Things a
Woman
Should Know
About Beauty

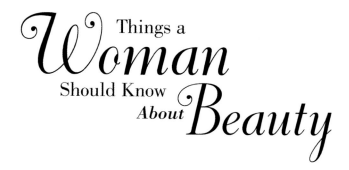

Things a **Woman** Should Know *About* Beauty

Karen Homer

PRION

First published in 2005.

This edition published in 2012 by
Prion
an imprint of the
Carlton Publishing Group
20 Mortimer Street
London W1T 3JW

10 9 8 7 6

ISBN 978-1-85375-830-0

A catalogue record of this book is available from the
British Library

Printed and bound in China

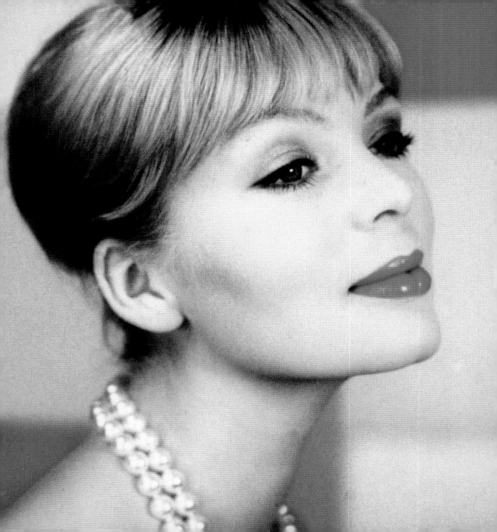

Contents

Introduction

*'Keep young and beautiful, it's your duty to be
beautiful, keep young and beautiful, if you want to
be loved'*

— Al Dubin and Harry Warren

A friend once told me her grandfather's descriptions of his
three daughters-in-law: one clever, one good and one
beautiful. Her mother was the clever one and we –
schooled in the Thatcher era – agreed that this was the
highest compliment. Neither of us admitted the truth:
forget clever, we wanted to be beautiful. I'm afraid being
good didn't even enter into the equation.

Possessing great beauty has been valued throughout history and, as we enter the twenty-first century, it is hard to imagine an age more obsessed by appearance. But what is beauty? Is it, as the old adage goes, in the eye of the beholder? It would be nice to think so, but most of us believe otherwise. Glossy magazines, advertising hoardings and Hollywood propaganda all push a (more often than not unrealistic) paradigm of beauty and, while most women don't aspire to look like some of the more waif-like and pre-pubescent models, few of us would turn down the genes that make Isabella Rosselini the icon of beauty that she is. Of course, having Ingrid Bergman for a mother obviously helps.

Admit it. You might never lay claim to being a great beauty but you want to make the best of yourself. You want to know how to put make-up on in ten minutes before the school run so it doesn't look as if you are wearing any, yet the permanent dark shadows under your eyes have miraculously disappeared. You want to be able to add a little more in the evenings without looking freakishly painted and feeling uncomfortably as if you are wearing a mask. Most of all you want to look like you, just a more beautiful version.

Genes aside, what are the tricks that transform a pretty girl into a 'great beauty'? How do you apply make-up and is there a cosmetic equivalent of 1960s bell-bottoms that you should avoid? How do you look after your skin when at the end of the day all you want to do is fall into bed, not apply a face-pack, and will giving up caffeine and dairy foods really make a difference to your complexion? What exactly is Botox and is it worth sacrificing your ability to raise your eyebrows for a smooth, unwrinkled forehead? What do you think about cosmetic surgery and where do you draw the line? Does being thin necessarily equal attractive and is it possible to break the mould and be big and beautiful?

This book answers these questions and more. It is for the woman who wants to know how to make the best of herself without losing the essence of what makes her individually attractive. Find out what to do if you feel naked without make-up but haven't changed your routine since you were sixteen. Discover how to look as if you've had a face-lift without actually having one – if only from the horror of unnecessary operations rather than occupying the moral high ground. Perhaps you are a serial dieter who is fed up with fads and fashions and just wants to find a sensible balance and learn which foods will make you glow from the inside... and how you can repair the damage done by one too many the night before. There are tricks to making yourself more beautiful, even if no one but you notices more than a subtle difference. After all:

'Nothing makes a woman more beautiful than the belief that she is beautiful'

— Sophia Loren

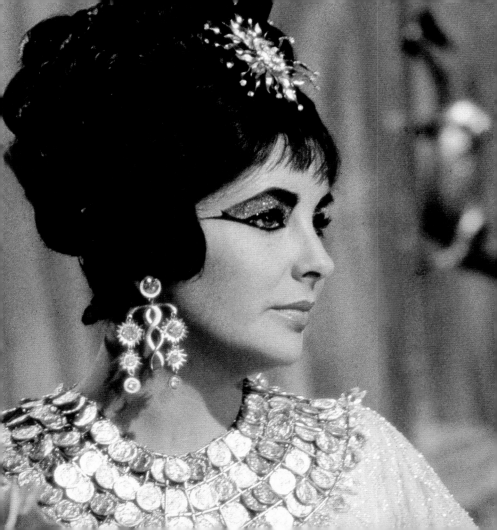

Painted Ladies

'A woman without paint is like food without salt'

— Plautus

Garishly painted faces on men and women alike covered the pock-marks and pimples of 18th-century aristocrats and red rouge and lipstick implied a healthy *joie de vivre*. But by the nineteenth century excessive make-up was seen as repulsive. Only the French continued to popularise the practice, earning them the reputation as people with something to hide.

Make-up has been around since Cleopatra painted her lips and elongated her eyes before setting off to seduce Mark Antony. The Ancient Egyptians wore foundation to lighten their skins as did the Greeks and Romans, who used white lead and chalk. Eyes were painted green, made from malachite, and outlined in black, derived from a sulphide of lead.

Pale has always been interesting as it showed women were affluent enough not to work outdoors. White faces were achieved by a variety of techniques: in the sixth century women bled themselves to maintain pallor, while from the Italian Renaissance through Elizabethan England lead paint was commonplace – the poisoning inflicted by this practice was an unfortunate side effect.

Making up has been a hazardous practice through the ages: belladonna – deadly nightshade – was used in the seventeenth and eighteenth centuries to dilate the eyes, thus simulating sexual arousal. It irrevocably damaged the eyesight.

Other dangerous ingredients had more devious effects. A certain Signora Toffana created an arsenic face powder for the women of rich Italian Renaissance families. They were strictly instructed never to ingest the powder themselves but to apply it when their husbands were around. Six hundred dead husbands – and many wealthy widows – later, Toffana was executed.

Victorians abhorred make-up, associating it with prostitutes, and even when it began to become fashionable again in the late nineteenth century it was a new natural look that gained popularity. Full make-up was seen as morally decadent if not downright sinful.

Not until the 1920s, when American women gained the vote and women's liberation spread, did make-up become popular again. Women showed their freedom to speak out with red lipstick, a social necessity.

Movie stars defined the make-up vogue throughout the 1930s, '40s and '50s, remaining heavy with varying accents on eyes, lips and face definition. The 1960s saw an explosion of experimentation with

Egyptian-style eyes and fantastical painted images such as butterflies. By the late 1970s things were toning down a little, although the 1970s and 1980s kept heavy eye make-up including an array of colourful eye-shadows and liners that make us cringe today. Not until the 1990s did the vogue for a more natural look return.

'Before she allows the world to judge her face, a woman is entitled to create it'

— Kennedy Fraser

As a potted history of make-up shows, we have come full circle. Heavy make-up is out, the natural look is in. Ironically the thing that most women want to learn about make-up is how to apply it so that it looks as if they aren't wearing any.

Starting from the base up is the question of how to make your skin look perfect, blemish free and youthfully translucent.

The answer is foundation – but only if you get it right.

Foundation means the foundation for the rest of your make-up. Foundation as in a base coat, not as in the foundation of houses, made from concrete. Some foundations are worryingly like concrete. Avoid them.

Foundation is designed to even out skin tones. That is your skin tone. The idea is not to paint on a skin tone you happen to like the colour of in the bottle. Wearing something that doesn't match your skin is a mask. It will crack – literally, if you apply as much as you will need of it to cover your own skin colour.

Foundation comes in liquids, gels, creams or solid sticks. It lays claim to light-reflecting pigmentation, extra luminosity and a finish of translucent silkiness.

A good foundation promises to bounce tiny light particles back off your skin to disguise everything from simple tiredness to fine lines, making it look younger and smoother. It promises equal brilliance in natural and artificial light.

Decent foundation will save you from an eternal greyness of complexion. No longer will you have to worry about bags, shadows, spots, rashes or blotchiness. You will be able to drink too much and sleep too little and get away with it.

And no one will know because the shades are so sophisticated that it won't look as if you are wearing make-up at all.

If only all this were true.

Foundation has developed in leaps and bounds since the orange paste of the past but it still needs careful choosing and correct application for it to really work.

First and most importantly, select a foundation that matches your skin tone exactly. That means exactly. Not approximately. And never go for a darker shade to try to look healthier or more tanned. It won't look convincing and you will have that tell-tale orange line across the base of your chin when you try to blend it.

In fact you will need a different foundation for winter and summer. If you are lucky you might only need foundation in winter or for full make-up when going out. This avoids lots of angst on summer holidays when you are in and out of the sea or pool.

Choose from a sheer formulation – for (genuinely) youthful or flawless skins – or a cream or compact version that will give more coverage. You will need to update regularly. Alas, a skin of 30 is not the same as one of 18.

Accept that as you get older you will probably want to wear more make-up, both to make you look better and

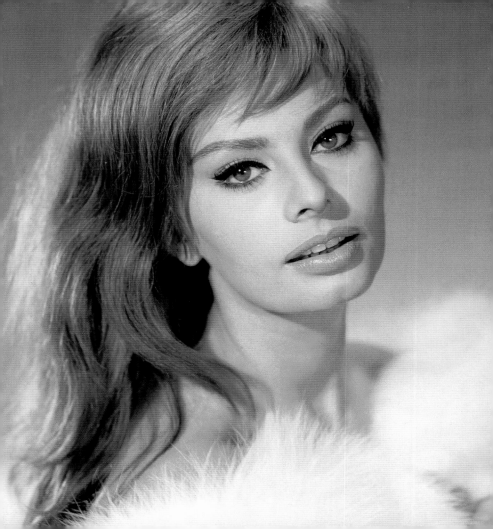

feel better. Accept, too, that as you get older make-up is more difficult to get right. Life is unfair.

When selecting your foundation, whatever your age, choose the lightest version you can. The aim is that you shouldn't look as if you are wearing foundation at all.

Iridescent versions sound wonderful but only for parties. Daytime wear will give you an alarming glitzy sheen that may not be quite the thing for the office. Even worse, pearlised foundations will highlight rather than disguise lines and wrinkles in natural light.

Don't wear foundation all the time and particularly not in the swimming pool, the gym or in bed – even if you are trying to impress a new lover. You will be caught out in the morning. Many love affairs have ended this way.

Wearing foundation at night is the cardinal sin of skincare. It will result in a Catch 22 situation: worse skin, more foundation needed. It will also leave a tell-tale stain on your bed-linen.

In fact, only when you are under 18 and spending an illicit night away are you allowed to fall asleep in full slap. After that, it will cost you both your complexion and your love life. No man is impressed with Coco the Clown the morning after the night before.

Application is as important as choice of shade. Unlike oilier versions many modern foundations apply quickly and evaporate. This gives you a matter of seconds to get the finish smooth and even. The pressure is on.

Apply moisturiser before foundation to give a good base to work on. Dot the foundation rather as if you are performing the sign of the cross – forehead, cheeks and chin. Use a sponge to work the foundation over the centre and out towards the edges of your face. Don't forget nostrils and over the ears.

You may wish to use concealer as well as foundation. This is invaluable for dark circles beneath the eyes. Dark circles are a fact of life past the age of 18, whatever you do.

Drinking gallons of water, getting plenty of sleep and arnica cream all help but unfortunately some of us are just destined to look as if we have gone a few rounds in the boxing ring. Nature is a cruel mistress.

There are certain times when even concealer won't cover dark circles – when you have a baby under the age of one, for example. Give yourself a break and resign yourself to this fact. Wear dark glasses instead.

If you are using concealer it goes on before foundation, not after. Dot the concealer sparingly before blending gently. Add a very little more if you need it, then apply foundation. Beware of loading concealer, foundation and powder beneath the eyes. It may look great for an hour but soon even the smallest wrinkles will be extra-defined in crêpey layers of make-up. Less is more.

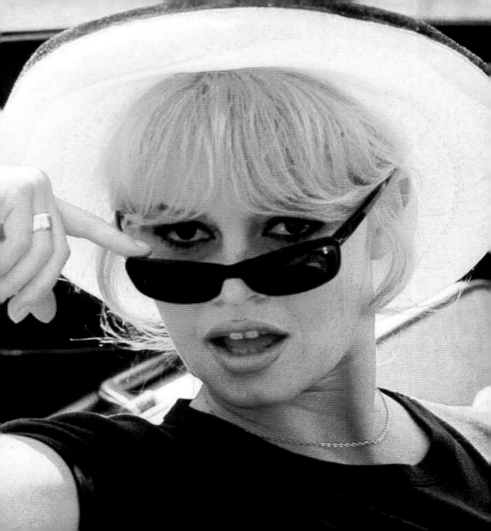

> Cotton buds were invented in 1923 by a Polish-born American named Leo Gerstenzang. Known by the brand name Q-Tips in the US, the Q stands for quality, the Tips refers to the cotton ends.

Concealer can be applied to blemishes with a brush or with a cotton wool bud or Q-Tip as they are known in the US.

Cosmetic – not talcum, for the beauty illiterate – powder is an optional extra that will finish and set your base. Again, choose a shade that matches your skin tone – and your foundation. You would be surprised how often the two don't work together.

Loose powders are thought superior and should be very sparingly applied with a brush. Blow the brush to remove excess first.

Start in the middle so that the shiny parts of your face get the most powder coverage. If you overdo it use a clean brush or cotton wool ball to remove the excess. It is worth reiterating – lines and wrinkles tend to collect powder. The trowel-load of make-up under the eyes look is not a good one.

Compact powders and powder puffs are messy and less effective than loose.

Loose powder is very messy, particularly when it upends itself inside your make-up bag. In fact any make-up spillages are horrendous. A bottle of foundation does not clean easily. Be careful.

An alternative is the hybrid between foundation and pressed powder. It looks like a compact but gives the coverage of a light foundation. It comes in one, easy-to-carry, not-so-breakable package that even fits in an evening bag.

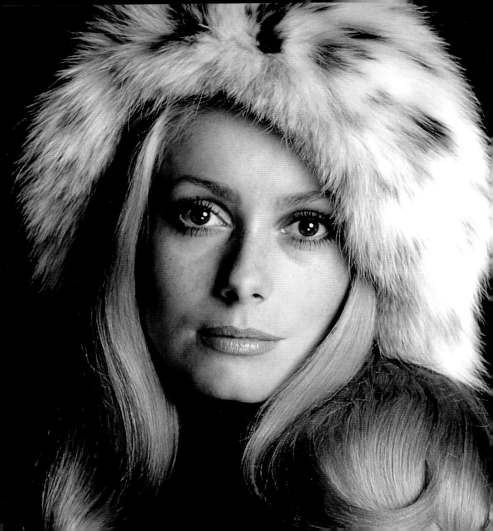

If you have reasonable skin to begin with, need only minimal coverage and the thought of a three-product base routine is too terrifying, this could be a good option for you – and it's cheaper.

Make-up artists do not like double compact powders as they claim that they don't give as good a finish as concealer, foundation and loose powder.

Real women love them because they solve the coverage problem in one hit and take a minute to apply instead of ten. Real women are not like make-up artists. They have lives that do not revolve around applying make-up.

Make-up artists are paid to give an immaculate finish and know how to achieve one. You are not a professional make-up artist. You are not being paid. Give yourself a break and make things easy – don't even try to emulate the glossy perfection of the magazine model.

Celebrities only look as good as they do when they go out because they employ professional make-up artists. This is a costly and high maintenance way to live. Luckily we are not expected to look as good as celebrities. Console yourself – a celebrity in close-up will look over-painted. They wear more make-up than looks good in real life because they need to look perfect in photographs.

Never wear this level of make-up unless you are being photographed – on your wedding day, for example. Don't do your wedding make-up yourself, employ a professional and listen to her. You will think you are wearing too much. You will not regret it when you see the photographs later.

Industry secret – lots of models have terrible skin. It's a chicken-and-egg situation: you need more make-up to cover the blemishes, therefore you get more spots from all the different products.

Nothing would be worse than having different make-up

artists work on you every day. The exposure to chemicals and oils found in such an array of make-up will play havoc with the finest of complexions.

Count yourself lucky you can choose make-up that suits your skin. Experiment accordingly – ask for oil-free make-up if you are prone to greasy skin and wear less if you do suffer from rashes or spots. They will not clear up if you plaster them with every product you can get your hands on.

Remember that make-up, like suncreams and perfumes, does not have an unlimited shelf-life. When the oil and pigment start to separate in a foundation you know it is time to throw it out.

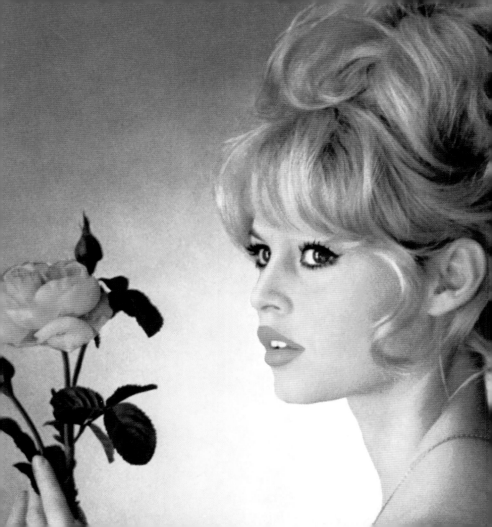

Cheek to Cheek

'From every blush that kindles in thy cheeks,
Ten thousand little loves and graces spring
To revel in the roses'

— Nicholas Rowe

Once you have evened out all the imperfections and given yourself a uniformly coloured face you might notice you look a little bland. The natural variations in your skin tone have been disguised and the delicate hint of healthy colour in your cheeks has disappeared. This is when to add the blusher.

If you haven't gone for the full plaster of Paris effect – and hopefully you haven't – you should still look like you and not a waxwork, but a little colour goes a long way to brightening up your face. If you do look like a waxwork, scrub off the lot and start again. A waxwork with rouged cheeks is about as bad as it gets.

Invest some time in choosing the right colour blusher as a good blusher is a make-up bag in itself. Apply it to lips and eyes as well as cheeks, finish with some basic lip-gloss and powder and a touch of mascara. Simple, yet elegant.

Some advise pinching your cheeks and copying your natural colour. Don't pinch too hard.

Blusher, like all types of make-up these days, is available in a confusing array of textures. Powder and cream are the two you are most likely to use. To apply powder blush first load your blusher brush – keep a brush separately for blusher, don't try to economise and double up on a translucent powder and blush brush, you will end up looking as if you have stuck your face in a pan of scalding water. The lobster effect is never attractive.

As with all things concerning make-up, less is more. Start slowly and build up if you don't think you have enough colour. Wipe the brush across your hand to get rid of excess – don't blow. Knowing your luck the colour will blow back and stick to your newly applied perfect finish foundation.

Few women really know where to apply blusher. The general rule with pink-peach tones is to highlight the apples of your cheeks, so start in the centre and work out to the edges. Avoid vertical up and down movements and stick to wide circles – stripes are for tigers.

Cream blusher is applied to the cheekbones. Use very sparingly, the colour is often more intense than you think and it's easier to add than take away. Blend downwards and outwards. Watch out for a tell-tale line where the blush finishes.

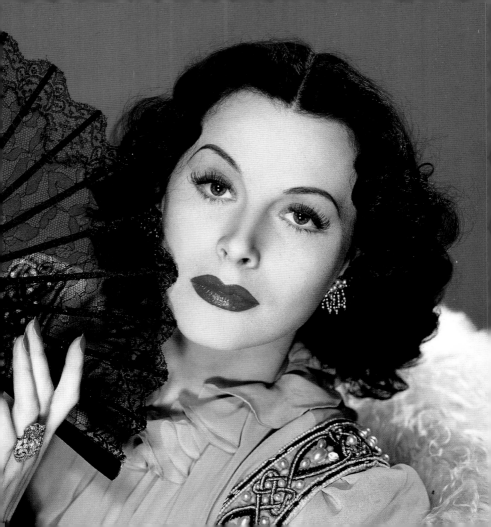

Blusher and highlighter are tricky to get right and look terrible when applied wrongly, hence the 'stick to the apples' rule, but there are a few tricks of the trade more specific to face shapes.

Heart-shaped: Highlight the cheekbones – the blusher goes on underneath, sweeping up towards the top of the ear. Be frugal.

Oval: Gentle shading only – trying to maximise cheekbones by using heavy blusher doesn't work.

Round or plump face: Make your face look thinner by shading the jawbone, the cheeks and the area just above the brow-bone. Avoid 1980s-style stripe of heavy blusher at all costs, however.

• 37 •

Square face: Soften by shading from jawline to cheeks and again on temples.

Broaden a pointed chin with blusher at the tip and highlighter above on either side.

Narrow a wide nose by highlighting the tip and sides.

For beauty modernists the latest product on the market is gel blusher. It is kind of a blush equivalent of lip gloss with less intense colour so it works well on freshly moisturised, nude faces. This is not the kind of blusher to use on top of full, heavy foundation. It won't have enough of an impact. And don't use it with loose powder as it has a shiny finish. You will risk ending up with a kind of home-made glue on your cheeks. Concentrate on the apples again for a youthful look.

It might be stating the obvious but this kind of make-up, designed for a youthful look, works best on youthful skins.

If you have shied away from blusher, prepare to meet a whole new you. It is the fastest route to comments on how well you look and if you apply it sparingly no one will ever know your secret. Blushing cheeks are the original marker of youth and innocence. In the words of the Bible:

'Blushing is the colour of virtue'

— Commentaries: Jeremiah iii

How wonderful that all our sins can be disguised by a simple dash of rose-pink powder.

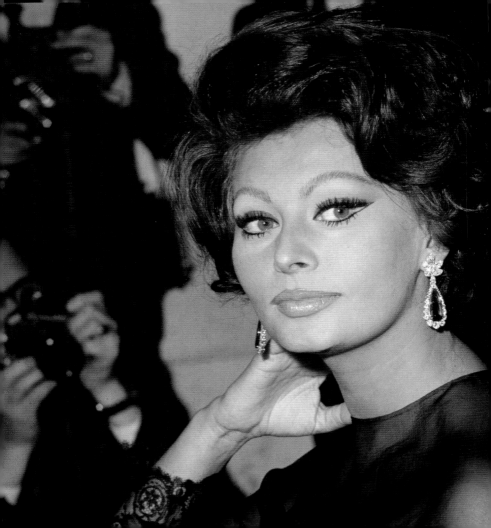

For Your Eyes Only

'The eyes like sentinels, hold the highest place in the body'

— Cicero

The amount of eye make-up you wear is a very individual choice, but almost every woman wears some, even if it is only a lick of mascara. Be warned – it is easy to make a faux pas when making up eyes.

This is partly because they are more subject to fashion than any other area of make-up and, as anyone who lived through the 1980s, drainpipe jeans, big shoulder pads, bigger hair and electric blue mascara will know, following fashion is not always a good thing.

Some of the worst: coloured mascara, electric blue, luminous green or thick with glitter, orange eye-shadow and matted clumps of lashes bound together by mascara applied so that it resembles tar.

Clear mascara is not so much a beauty mistake as a pointless creation. Why? It doesn't even hold your lashes in place for long, has no thickening or colouring properties and yet for a short while in the late 1980s women seem to think it is was the answer to their prayers for more natural make-up.

More embarrassing still are first attempts at plucking your eyebrows – full gorilla to whippet-thin in one over-frenzied session with the tweezers, permanent stubble as you try to rein in the re-growth or the bizarre trend for shaving a patch from the middle of your eyebrow – we have all lived them. Burn the photos and start again.

As you can see, getting eye make-up right is tricky. There is more to it than meets the eye, if you'll excuse the pun. It is even trickier because you tend to want different weights for different occasions and different stages in life. Learning to apply it in your late teens is all very well but not if you are still doing the same thing 20 years later.

There is as much paraphernalia dedicated to applying eye make-up as there is to performing a minor surgical operation. Eye pencil, crayon, mascara, pearly eyeshadow, matt eyeshadow, cream eyeshadow, highlighter pencil, brow-defining pencil, eyelash curlers, eyelash comb, tweezers, sponge applicator and brushes – at least three different weights.

Don't be afraid. Much of this is unnecessary.

Minimal emphasis: For a really natural look, apply a pale neutral colour over the entire lid. One with a light sheen works well. Next, apply a slightly darker shade along the crease of your lid. Brush this same colour through your brow for maximum effect and finish with a single coat of mascara. On many people very dark brown is softer and more natural than black.

More definition: Use a pale shadow over the lid, then a liquid eyeliner to paint a fine line along your upper lashes. Flick the line slightly upward at the edge to lift the eye shape. This takes practice so if you look like Cleopatra on a bad day start again. On the whole, mistakes are best remedied by starting all over again but repeated attempts will leave your eyes red and watery – never a good look. Instead, a cotton bud dipped in eye-make-up remover can be very gently used to sheer the line down to narrow perfection. Finish with one coat of mascara but curl your eyelashes and define your brows with a pencil.

Full on face: Use foundation on your lids if you are going to apply a great deal of eye make-up. It is a better base than powder. But, before starting, brush some translucent

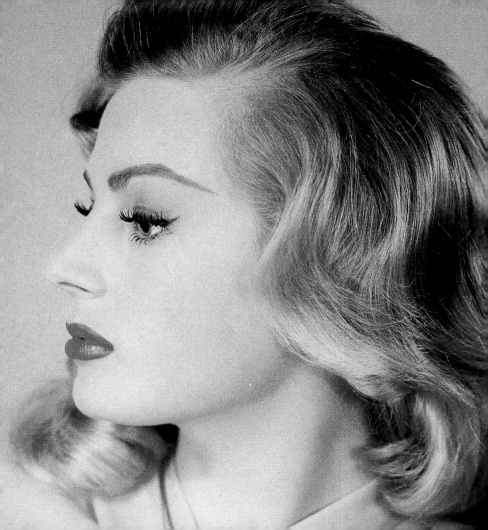

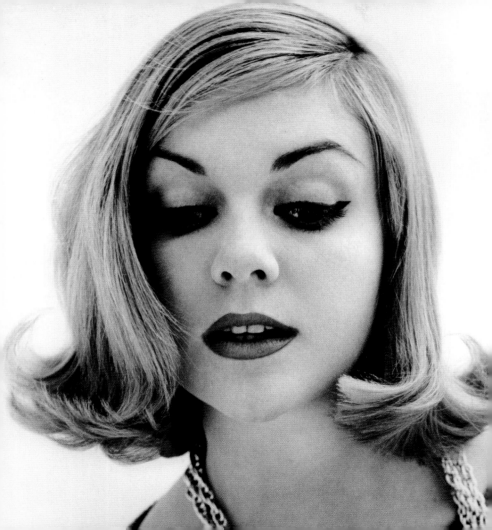

powder beneath the lids – this will act as a safety net, catching any loose particles of eye make-up, and can be swept up afterwards.

Use a mid-tone eye-shadow – mid-grey, taupe or even plum work well for a more dramatic evening look – all over the lid. Using a small brush apply the same colour along the lower lid as close as you can. Don't blink. Clean the brush before blending the outer edges of this line. Take a darker but similar shade of shadow and trace along the upper lid. Blend into the paler base.

Accentuate the eyes with dark liquid liner on the upper lid. Flick the line out a little more. Be bold – feline eyes are seductive. But don't get carried away or you will look as if you have had bad cosmetic surgery. Lastly, brush a highlighter shade across your brow-bone. Define the brows with pencil or shadow and apply two coats of mascara to both top and bottom lids. Comb through to separate lashes.

Eyebrows: If only making up the eyes was only about, well, making up the eyes. Unfortunately eyebrows are, as one make-up artist put it, the pillars of the face. Any cracks and the whole effect will come crashing down.

Neatening up your eyebrows is one of the fastest ways to change the appearance of your face. It can be so effective that you barely need apply make-up at all to receive flattering comments. But beware. Don't try to radically change the shape of your brows – rather like drastic plastic surgery it is better to work with what you have got. Think tidying up rather than rebuilding.

Over-zealous plucking will leave you looking peculiarly surprised. Remember those warnings about the wind changing and leaving you stuck with one expression. And before you say, oh well, they'll grow back… they might not!

General advice is to concentrate on the hairs below the brow as it is the top of the brow that gives your face

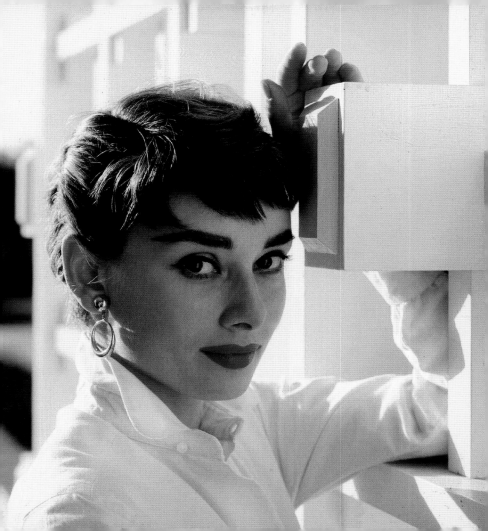

definition. Before you give a final pull, draw the hair back with your tweezers and see if you really can do without it. The aim is to open up the eye area, so removing hairs across the bridge of the nose is a good idea. Don't overdo it – if you genuinely do feel as if you have one long caterpillar of an eyebrow snaking across your face it is perhaps worth getting a professional to do your plucking the first time, then you can just keep it up.

Take heart – apparently even supermodel Gisele has eyebrows that are too close together.

It is a good idea to get a professional to pluck your eyebrows at least once. It is surprising how different you will look. Then you just have to do general maintenance. Over-plucking or breaking hairs are the worst amateur mistakes.

Top make-up artist tricks to deaden pain: an ice-cube, although it might be said that freezing your face is painful enough in itself, baby teething gel or a dab of clove oil. Only bother if you have a really low pain threshold – no gain without a little pain.

Insiders don't pluck at all but have their eyebrows threaded. Threading, a practice that originated in Asia and seems virtually impossible to master, is hard to come by. It is an extraordinary experience. The practitioner – small, unimposing and looking as if she has the wisdom of hundreds of years of female intuition locked inside her – takes a cotton thread and holding it between her hand and teeth it flies about your brow, catching and pulling without pain until, before you know it, you are transformed. Unfortunately, this is the kind of highly skilled technique that few can master. Done badly it is worse than not at all.

Waxing is a terrible idea. It is almost impossible to get the kind of precision you need.

There is no such thing as a fashionable eyebrow. You might think there is when you see models' brows go from virtually not there to as bushy as a broom-head apparently in the space of weeks (heartening to know that these girls are as hairy as the rest of us) but brow shape is as individual as face shape. It all comes down to what suits your bone structure. So don't copy a magazine.

If you over-pluck – and who hasn't? – use an eye-shadow and eye pencil to shade in the gaps. Not ideal but better than looking like a patch of newly sown grass that hasn't quite taken.

Talking of over-lush vegetation around the eyes – a note about false eyelashes. Don't.

Well, do if you are going to a 1960s revival Biba party but otherwise this is as dated a beauty look as you can get. Anyway, do you really want to be fussing around with all that glue... and what if one falls off into your cocktail?

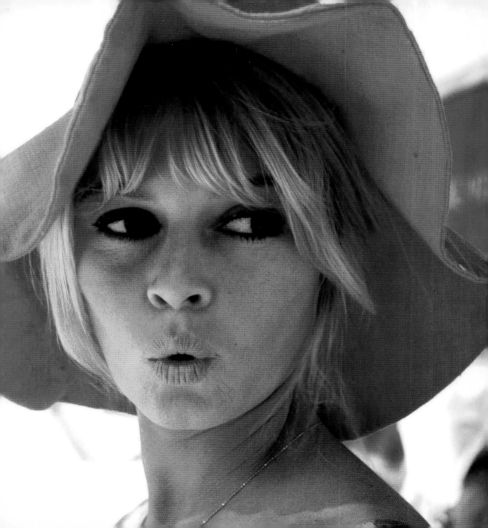

Life is enough of a farce without adding to your problems.

Similar caveats when making up the eye area: fantasy. Forget butterflies, flowers or graffiti-type creations unless you are appearing in a Galliano couture catwalk show. Chances are you are not.

A word about colour. If you do want to use a strong colour on your eyes it is even more important that you apply it well. Loose powders are densest in pigment so provide the most intense colour. Creamier pressed eyeshadows may appear intense in the compact but look far less so when applied to the skin. Don't be tempted to apply more for a deeper colour – you'll just end up with an uneven oil slick of colour that is impossible to blend.

The only colours that endure are neutrals in shades from pale honey to dusky brown, variations on grey and at a push, varieties of plum... not emperor purple but a berry colour, please. Wear orange, blue or green to costume parties only.

Glitter is a tricky one – some iridescent shadows are nice for the evening but glitter applied randomly to your lids will flake, making you look as if you have spent the day at a child's birthday party. Of course, if you have spent the day at a child's birthday party and are covered in glitter you can always pretend it was intentional. (Hands-on fathers beware, men in glitter is a bad thing.)

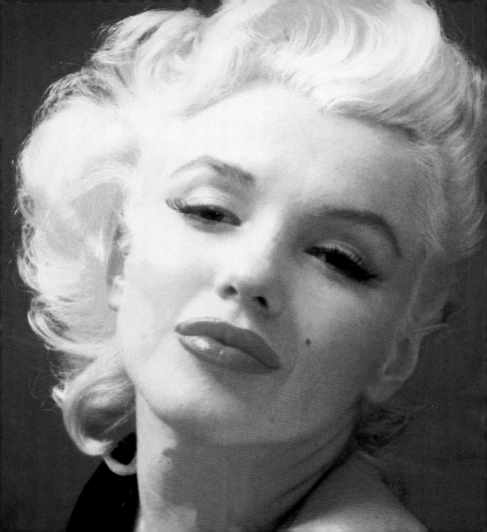

Just One Kiss

'Where lipstick is concerned, the important thing is not colour, but to accept God's final word on where your lips end'

— Jerry Seinfeld

Lipstick. Love it or hate it, it is the one piece of make-up that every woman has tried. All small girls (and some boys) have tried it too, as any mother will tell you when she finds her favourite Chanel lipstick smeared all over the bedroom walls.

Even if you wear nothing else a lick of lipstick will brighten up your face. Chosen well it can give the illusion that you are

Lipsticks first appeared five thousand years ago. It is said that Cleopatra's lipsticks were made from finely crushed carmine beetle to make a deep red pigment. This was then mixed with ants' eggs to form a lipstick. In Elizabethan times lipsticks were made from a blend of cochineal and beeswax.

During the Second World War the ends of used lipsticks were collected and melted together and re-solidified. Women had on average two new lipsticks to last the five-year duration of the war. When lipstick ran out solid rouge was used on lips.

wearing everything else as well. Chosen badly it can make your skin tone several shades poorer, your eyes recede into your face and render your clothes so badly matched that you appear colour blind. Apply it badly and you will look as if you have had a nasty accident with a broken glass bottle.

Finding the perfect lipstick colour is akin to searching for the Holy Grail.

If you do ever find it there is every probability that it will be discontinued that same month. Life is like that.

A woman needs at least three lipsticks in her make-up bag. One for day, one for night and one for emergencies: fire-engine red. And before you start on the righteous indignation feminist bandwagon remind yourself that strong red lipstick is not tarty; it is classic 1950s stylish. Therefore, it works best with classic 1950s-style clothes. Worn with mini-skirts and stilettos red lipstick is tarty. Moreover, it should be applied perfectly; the slightest slip is sluttish in the extreme.

Lipstick draws attention to the mouth and colours the lips in a way that mimics sexual arousal. Or so the theory goes. It is unfortunate that lipstick is seen as an essential tool of seduction but is the worst thing to wear when you are kissing.

Luckily few men seem to mind and there is something delightfully old-fashioned about retiring to the Ladies to repair your lipstick and of course powder your nose. This shouldn't be a euphemism if you want to look good all night.

If you do choose to wear heavy make-up, keep it looking good and touched up with regular trips to the mirror. It's more vain to assume you are still looking good than to check. A slipped 'face' or a smeared mouth is not attractive. No matter how many martinis you have drunk there is no excuse. Bear this in mind when you decide to put on full slap. It can be more trouble than it is worth.

Back to lipstick – for daywear you need a neutral. Your choice will depend on your skin tone so you will probably need a different shade for summer and winter.

As far as neutrals go, brown- or beige-pink-based shades are the most successful. Lip glosses offer more shine, less colour but have an appealing dewy naturalness about them. They do, however, only last a matter of minutes before you need to reapply.

Some experts recommend a touch of lip balm or treatment cream to stop lipstick running and keep it looking fresh. Others recommend powder on the lips to even out the surface. Contradictory advice means one thing: try it for yourself. A dot of Vaseline might seem to work but very waxy balms will coagulate taking half your lip colour with them. Flecks of peeling lip are bad enough but lipstick-coloured ones are a whole other embarrassment. A soft lip cream left for a few minutes to thoroughly sink in is your best bet.

Emphasising your lips requires lip pencil. Anyone who thinks lip pencil is a waste of money if you are buying lipstick, think again. Blurry edges are one step away from looking like a naughty child who has had their fingers in the jam jar.

That said, don't just buy one lip pencil and use it with every shade of lipstick you have. They have to match. Yes, it is expensive, but if a job is worth doing…

Once the lipstick is defined you shouldn't be able to see the pencil – it just gives a sharp edge. I was once told to colour my whole lips in with the pencil to create an evenly coloured base before putting on my lipstick. I think this is why I spent so many years chewing the lipstick off my lips as they flaked in protest.

A lip brush is by far and away the easiest route to good, even lip colour. Look closely at the finish achieved by those women who apply lipstick while driving the car, without a mirror on the train etc. and console yourself that it isn't worth mastering the art as it never looks perfect. Who wants to be able to apply lipstick by holding it in their cleavage *à la* Molly Ringwald in *The Breakfast Club*, anyway?

Fill in your whole lip area, right up to the lip line, work into the corners – you might not look at yourself with your mouth open but anyone you speak to does.

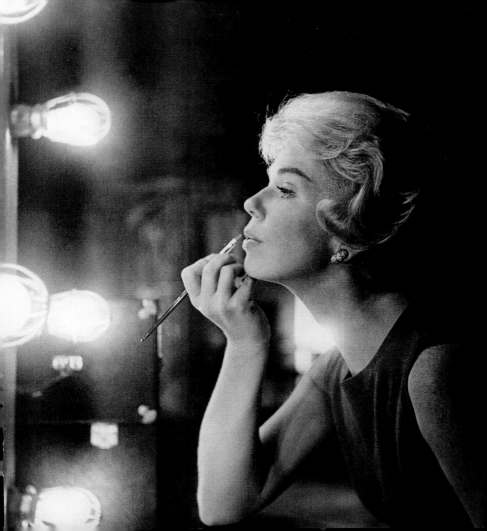

Blot your lips with tissue to fix the colour and add another layer of colour or gloss for maximum density. Don't apply powder as a fixative. It will dull the colour and give you a dusty mouth.

Ultra-glossy lips are the one time when you might want a blurrier edge, so don't use liner. Do make absolutely sure that there are no rogue bits of dry skin by scrubbing lips first – exfoliant or a toothbrush with a little lipsalve on it are equally effective. Scrub hard enough and your lips will end up so red you won't need lipstick at all. Joke.

Apply colour first if you wish or gloss straight from the pot with your fingers. Don't overdo it unless you want to look like a *Baywatch* babe. Well, if you are sure.

It is possible to slightly change the shape of your lips by emphasising lower or upper lips, bows, etc. with your lip pencil. Do not, I repeat, do not try to give yourself a full pout if you have thin lips. Drawing a false lip line well outside your own never works. Maybe for two minutes in front of the mirror in fake lighting you might convince yourself but in natural light, seen from the side or after anything to eat or drink, you will look like a drag queen after a hard night on the town.

It is easier to reduce the appearance of a full mouth by outlining just within the edge of the lips and colouring in a shade lighter – rosy shades work well on full lips. The same goes for wide lips: outline with a dark pencil and fill in with a very slightly lighter lipstick and blend. Don't wear the classic attention-drawing gloss or shine – these are all designed to make lips look bigger and fuller.

Why would anyone want to minimise full lips when Julia Roberts and collagen implants are the beauty paradigm? Take it from someone with a perfect, 1920s small rosebud mouth. We live in an era of wide-mouthed princesses.

A few things to worry about when you are wearing heavy make-up that might convince you to keep it for special occasions only...

For most women, it may not be worth putting in a huge amount of time and effort every day. A dab of foundation or powder to even out the complexion, some concealer beneath the eyes and a dash of lipstick to brighten up your face takes up the few minutes you have to spare in the mornings. Trying to make yourself look like someone else is not the aim, particularly when it means a day of worrying that your true face will be revealed. Consider the following:

Heavy rain when you have forgotten your umbrella.

Wiping your hand across your face or rubbing your eyes, forgetting your new and carefully applied make-up regime. Or worse still someone reaches out their hand saying 'you just have a little mark here, let me wipe it off' and in one sweep your 'face' has been displaced by a few millimetres or simply has an irreparable hole in it.

Kissing people on the cheek and leaving a tell-tale mark.

Carrying a baby to whom noses and cheeks represent the biggest playthings ever, particularly when put in their mouth. Saliva is a surprisingly effective make-up remover.

Forgetting your make-up bag and being stuck somewhere without the tool kit to repair any damage.

Save your full camouflage for when you really need it and when people comment on how great you look don't think 'God, I must look awful the rest of the time'. Think how nice it is to be complimented when you have made an effort.

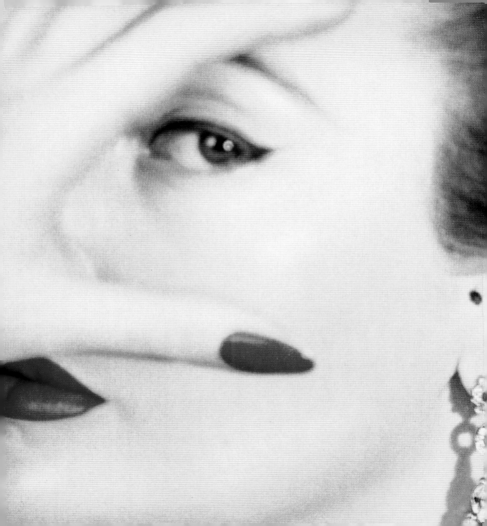

Get it Nailed

Faces aren't the only part of you that beauty addicts deem should be painted. Once you start thinking about how much people can tell about you from the state of your nails you will be dialling the manicurist before you know it. Everything from overall health, vitamin and mineral deficiencies, a propensity to neuroses or a keen interest in gardening are easy to spot from simply looking at a person's hands. A set of ragged nails nibbled to the quick can ruin the appearance of a beautiful woman and betray her hidden insecurities.

A week later, when you realise quite how much work it takes to maintain perfect nails – not to mention the restrictions on your lifestyle – you will throw your hands up in the air and resign yourself to small imperfections. The only women who have perfect nails are hand models... or wealthy (bored) ladies who lunch.

When you start weeping over a torn nail you know that your priorities have become a little warped.

Nails grow on average about 4 mm a month, faster during spring, summer and pregnancy. Young people's nails grow faster than old people's and stress or illness can slow down or even stop growth. Ridges, splitting or flaking nails and white specks all indicate ill health, and anaemia can be diagnosed from colourless nails.

Perfect talons are a hindrance to everyday life. They make everyday tasks such as opening drawers or dialling telephones difficult, they catch on loose threads and scratch your children as you pick them up. The cliché of the secretary filing her nails at her keyboard becomes even more absurd when you realise quite how difficult it is to type with long fingernails.

Long nails are quite useful for picking out splinters or scratching things off surfaces but they are not designed for this and are likely to break, which kind of defeats the object.

If you ever want long, perfect nails for a special occasion, use fake ones. But have them done professionally and resist the temptation to keep them on until they fall off of their own accord. Acrylic nails can damage the nail beneath if they are not applied correctly.

• 71 •

Try to resist the temptation to use false nails while your real ones are growing in. If you are too embarrassed to reveal the state of your nails and do want to use fake ones make sure you keep the nails beneath well moisturised. When you take off the falsies the new growth will be nice and strong.

Massaging your nails with olive oil works as well as investing in expensive (and in very small bottles) specialist nail oil.

File your nails once a week with a fine emery board (preferably not a coarse board and NEVER a steel file – this is like exfoliating your skin with a Brillo pad) just to keep the edges from splitting. Nails split just like hair and we have our hair cut regularly to maximise healthy growth. The same goes for nails.

The kind of nails we all should aspire to are moderate and uniform in length, nicely shaped and white, topping off smooth, unblemished hands. Practical and good-looking, what more could you ask for?

Gardeners and cooks should definitely keep their nails short. So should anyone who has less than healthy nails.

A love of gardening does not necessarily spell the kiss of death to good-looking nails and hands. You can rub a bar of soap over your nails to protect the cuticle – make sure you get it beneath your nails and you won't have to dig out dirt for days afterwards – apply a layer of hand cream or simply wear gloves.

Remove layers of dead skin from hands with an exfoliant and moisturise afterwards.

Household remedies for hands: exfoliate with oatmeal or salt and Vaseline. Use lemon juice to remove dirt or to bleach discoloured, nicotine-stained fingers and sugar mixed with vegetable oil to remove ink or oil stains.

A once-a-week (or more likely, once-a-month) miracle cure for rough hands is covering your hands with moisturiser,

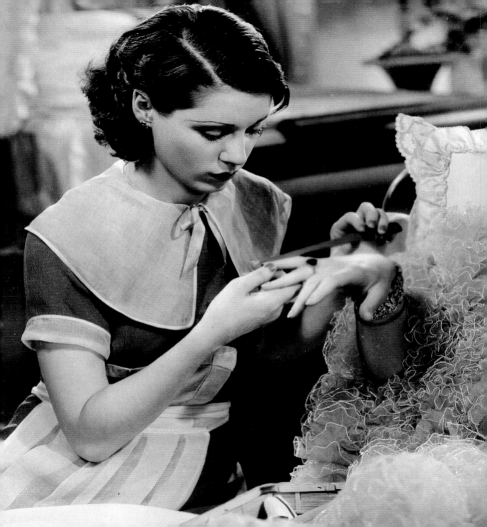

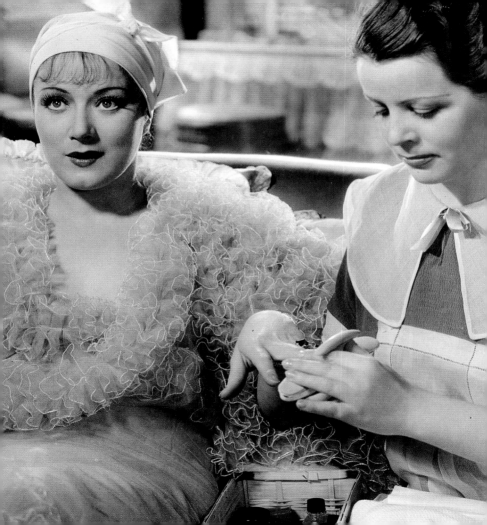

slipping them into a pair of disposable gloves and leaving them on all night. Wake up to skin soft as a baby's bottom and – if you wriggle in your sleep – some very sticky bedclothes.

Like all things to do with cosmetics the more artificial products you apply, the more likely you are to damage your nails (just like hair and skin). This is particularly true of nail polish and remover that contain acetone, which makes nails very dry. Try to find a remover that doesn't contain it.

Washing detergents and household chemicals have the same effect. Better get used to those Marigolds.

If you follow all these tips you might stand a fighting chance of having a decent set of nails. Then you can have some fun with colour.

Perfectly painted nails are best done by professionals but if you have a steady hand (accept that if you are right-handed the nails done by your left may not be so perfect and vice-versa) and a spare half hour you can do a manicure yourself.

Bear in mind that you can do very little after your manicure until your nails dry and fully harden and that can take hours. Before you say 'fine, I've got the evening to myself', think of undoing the buttons of your jeans to go to the loo, uncorking the bottle of wine you need to enjoy your evening of pampering, dialling your best girlfriend, etc.

How to manicure – the full experience

Remove old polish: ALWAYS remove old polish. The best way is by using a cotton pad soaked in remover and holding it to the nails for a minute or so to let it absorb the polish before wiping off. This stops dark polishes bleeding all over your fingers, which completely undermines attempts to make your hands look good.

Cuticles: Apply cuticle cream. Soak fingers in warm soapy water for five minutes. Dry thoroughly. Push back cuticle gently with a cuticle stick designed for the job, not the nearest sharp implement and certainly not the fingernails on your other hand. Trim hangnails with cuticle clippers.

Shaping nails: Only use scissors if you are taking considerable length off your nails, otherwise just file. The jury is out on scissors versus clippers – some experts believe clippers cause cracks. Cut from edge to centre either side for a rounded shape, straight across for square. Shape with a file once the length has gone, similarly from edge to centre at an angle of approximately 45 degrees. File the tip by holding the file vertically and filing downwards.

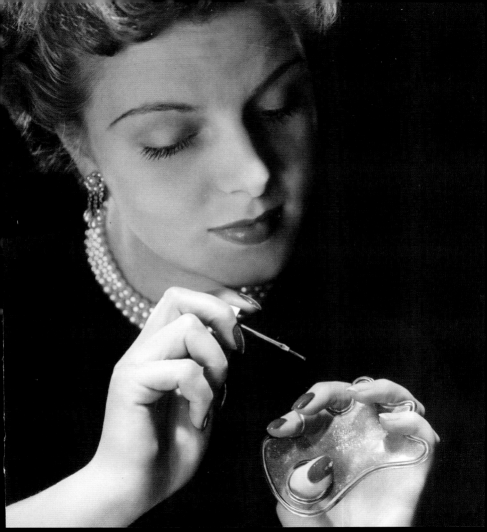

Pointed, round or square: Square nails are more utilitarian and good if you want to balance practicality with looks. Rounded nails are more elegant in a 1950s kind of way. Perfect for holding champagne glasses and applying bright red lipstick in an ostentatious fashion. Whatever you decide make sure they are all the same length. No nail, no matter how long it has taken you to grow or how proud you are of your achievement, is worth hanging onto if the others are all shorter.

Buff and colour: A good buff and a lick of clear polish (or none at all) are fine for a natural, healthy look. Otherwise a base coat, two coats of colour and a top coat are usual for the hardiest manicure. Choose bright colour only if you have elegant hands and long, well-shaped fingers. Nothing looks worse than a smudge of fire-engine red on the end of potato fingers.

Paint from bottom to top vertically, never across the nail horizontally. Use a good-quality brush and don't overload it. Don't paint too near the cuticle or you will flood it and look as if you have had a nasty accident. Three strokes should do one coat.

Repairs: Torn nails can be glued with specialist nail glue if you catch them quickly. Remove polish first, apply glue sparingly and buff once it has hardened. Use nail strengthener on top for maximum longevity.

Chipped polish can be painted over carefully in a dab-dab fashion. Use quick dry or a hair-dryer if you are late for an important date. Otherwise leave alone as quick dry can dull the finished effect.

Once you have done your manicure sign off for the rest of the day. Lay your hands on a silken cushion and have someone feed you grapes as you recline enjoying a foot massage. If only...

How to manicure – the lazy way

Remove old polish: No getting away from it.

Moisturise: Apply oil or lotion to nails and round the edges.

File: Give a once over with a file. Try to remember to go from edge to centre. Don't panic if nails aren't perfect.

Paint: Use a neutral or pale colour if you have fudged the shaping a bit. Or leave naked and just apply some more hand-cream. At least this way you don't need to wait for them to dry.

Dry: You can use quick dry but don't make a habit of it. Professionals' tip is to wait until your nails are touch dry and then run under icy cold water.

How not to apply polish...

If you are the kind of lazy, sluttish girl who simply whacks a new layer of polish on top of the old (particularly tempting in summer when unpainted toenails are too ugly but time is too scarce) re-read the previous section immediately. And broken nails cannot be held in place by a concrete layer of old polish – your sins will catch up with you eventually when the whole lot lifts off the evening you are showing off your new Jimmy Choos at a party.

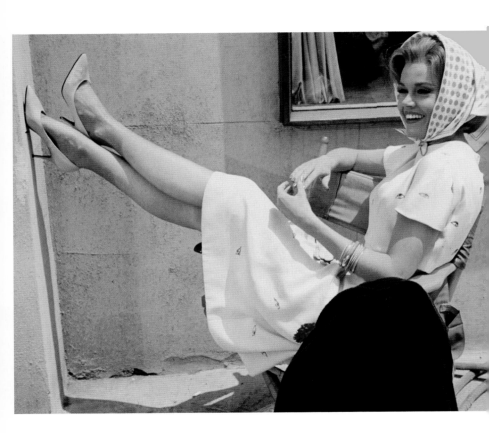

Best Foot Forward

'My feet, they haul me round the house,
They hoist me up the stairs;
I only have to steer them, and
They ride me everywheres'

— Frank Gelett Burgess

Feet: now there's an ugly word in the beauty industry. Few of us pay enough, if any, attention to our feet. Horny old toenails, yellowing pads of rough and flaky old skin and that's before we start on the warts and corns, untended blisters and lurking fungi that would rival the dampest of woodland grottos.

It is amazing how many women who paint their faces to perfection, scrub the cellulite from their thighs and spend a fortune on anti-ageing creams neglect their feet. Until summer, when poor harried feet are expected to metamorphose into smooth, elegant and entirely un-knobbly appendages that set off a pair of designer micro-sandals to perfection.

No chance. If you don't look after your feet year round they will not forgive you quickly.

There are three experts you need for perfect feet: the chiropodist, the podiatrist and the pedicurist. These do, of course, overlap depending on whether you are treating your feet for health or vanity.

Health is, of course, relative. If you have really neglected your feet go to a professional now. A chiropodist will sort our your corns and bunions, have the dead skin razored off and check you have no hidden nasties just waiting to spread. (Bear in mind that a simple pedicure can spread something that has been lurking in your little toenail across the whole foot and that takes some getting rid of.)

Don't try tackling corns yourself as you will do far more harm than good.

Similarly, the podiatrist will deal with deformities – looking at the foot from a structural point of view. And before you dismiss the idea ask yourself if you are in pain from walking in the wrong shoes, if your toes look as if they are bending the wrong way, or if your insteps seem a little too arched or have simply fallen flat?

A word about shoes: shoes need to be supple at the front to allow movement and hard enough at the back to give good ankle support. Slip your hand inside and make sure you can't feel any hard seams or dramatic arches.

Needless to say, all desirable shoes – 4-inch stilettos, tiny strappy sandals, anything from Manolo Blahnik – fall

The average person will walk around 100,000 miles in a lifetime, taking 8,000 to 10,000 steps a day. Each step you take can exert a pressure on your feet that equals three or four times your body weight. During an average walking day this can equal a force of hundreds of tons. Uneven pressure from ill-fitting shoes or high heels will lead to the formation of calluses and hard skin.

outside this category except for those soft-as-can-be, kid leather driving shoes that cost as much as a year's worth of pedicures. And I wouldn't count on them offering much foot support either.

But it is amazing how much your feet will let you get away with and if there are no major problems other than having

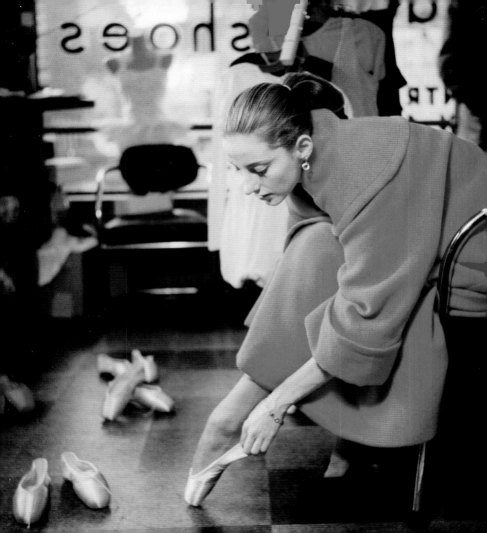

let your feet look after themselves for too long consult the pedicurist. The scraping and cutting may be almost as good as a chiropodist but the focus will be on the nails.

The thought of having a pedicure but not having your toes painted seems rather absurd. That is the whole point, isn't it? Not always. An expert pedicurist should be able to make your feet look as good *au naturel* as they would finely painted.

And if you feel cheated that you are paying for such a subtle difference ask for a foot massage in the time it would usually take to paint the nails.

Nail polish is not great for your nails (on a par with coating them in plastic). But classic Chanel red toenails are a beauty necessity when it comes to looking chic in high summer.

A word on colour: This particular Chanel red is the only enduringly stylish colour for toenails. A muted coral pink or beige comes a close second but better to leave your nails nude and buff them perfectly.

Colours such as the cult *Pulp Fiction* Rouge Noir with all its imitators come and go. Keep up to date to avoid looking hopelessly out of vogue. There is never an excuse for blue nail polish.

Strike a balance: have your toes painted for a few months of the year and let them rest through the winter. Except for one-off special Christmas parties of course. There is nothing more satisfying than parading a pair of perfect feet in the middle of winter.

Note: fire-engine red on toenails classy, on fingernails tarty.

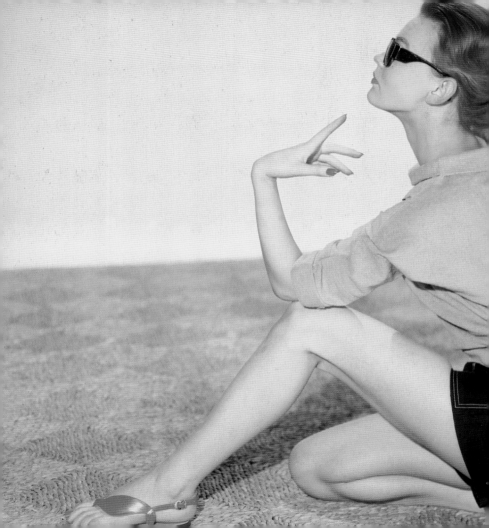

DIY pedicure

Even if you don't go the whole hog at least give your feet the benefit of regular attacks with a pumice stone (or hard metal remover) to stop the build-up of dry skin.

Soak your feet first in warm soapy water – add some bath salts for maximum therapeutic effect. Relax for a while (minutes easily turn into hours, although a tepid foot-spa isn't all that appealing). Dry thoroughly - as your mother always told you - behind your ears and between your toes. Obviously ears are nothing to do with pedicures but when it comes to the proverbial growing of cabbages comparisons can be made.

Rub off dead skin, smooth with a foot file and finish with your preferred cream, lotion or even a pure vegetable oil. Heels and big toes are the worst offenders for hard patches. (Accept that you get – and need – more hard patches in summer to protect bare feet. Hence the agony of blisters even in well-worn sandals the first time you wear them.)

Toenails

Clip toenails straight across – not down the sides as this can promote infection. File as per fingernails if you care about a really neat finish.

Apply cuticle cream, push back cuticles. Use exfoliating cream to smooth feet, rinse and dry… thoroughly! Finish with lotion.

Separate your toes with a length of loo roll wound round your toes, cotton balls or if you have such a thing a foam or rubber toe separator. (If you do own such a thing you probably don't need to be reading this section.)

Apply base coat, two layers of colour and top coat as per fingernails. Leave to dry as long as possible before putting socks or shoes back on – preferably overnight.

Some pedicurists will assure you that if you apply some oil

to the nails, wrap your feet in cling film and then put your socks back on the polish will last. This worked for me once – the other time I took off my socks only to be greeted with a blood bath – and a wasted pedicure.

Wander barefoot wearing just a silk negligée and take great pleasure in admiring your perfectly painted feet. Accessorise with a handsome man and an expensive bottle of champagne.

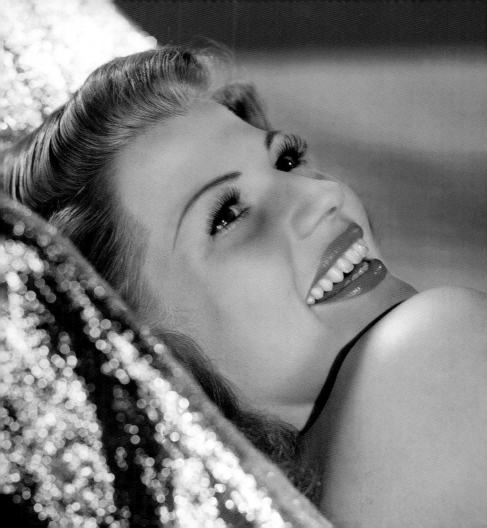

Pearly Whites

'My, what big teeth you have, Mr Wolf'

— Little Red Riding Hood

People notice teeth – well, very good or very bad teeth at least. As soon as you open your mouth, before you have even said anything, the impression you give is changed.

There was a time when you accepted the teeth you were born with, a little crooked, a little yellowing over time, your gnashers were there to do precisely that – grind your food. Alas, no more. A Day-Glo white smile is seen as the new fast track to youthful good looks. No longer the preserve of Hollywood actresses and toothpaste models you are as likely to be blinded by your bank manager when he shakes your hand and smiles. Enough to put you off paying back that loan.

Talking of loans, you might need one to have any of the cosmetic dentistry available these days, as it doesn't come cheap. We're talking thousands, not hundreds, of pounds.

Bleaching, veneers, anterior and direct composites, ceramic crowns, fibre-reinforced composite bridges, indirect porcelain, composite inlays and onlays, anterior crowns, micro-abrasion treatment... the list goes on.

So where do you draw the line? Basic orthodontic treatment is very commonplace for children. (You know something is considered a necessity when you can get it on the National Health Service.) Increasingly, braces are common on adults too. When celebrities – think Cher and Tom Cruise – start showing a mouth full of metal you know something has changed, although somehow the stigma of teenage train-tracks will always endure. And how about those first kisses with the boy next door and your eternal dread that you would lock braces?

If you wear braces now rest assured that – apparently – they are considered a fashion statement. After all, nothing is as unfashionable as being seen not to care about how you look.

The Americans are the first to tell you that they can spot a British actor a mile off – he hasn't had his teeth fixed. And by Hollywood standards that is bleached an improbable shade of white and lined up in a way that would impress the most pedantic of draughtsmen.

Braces aside, there are other ways of quickly and painlessly – orthodontics take months if not years and when they tighten those braces it hurts – straightening teeth. A veneer or cap will cover gaps and straighten small imperfections in, for example, front teeth. A veneer is usually less intrusive as it simply involves sticking moulded porcelain onto the roughened surface of your existing tooth. A cap involves filing the edges of the tooth down to form a narrow shape onto which the artificial cap can be fitted. It cannot be securely welded onto the original tooth without significant filing down – not a pretty sight if you lose it.

Beware of a mouthful of capped teeth if you hope to make an impression at night. Ultra-violet light will render them black! Not such a good look if you are hoping to get lucky in a nightclub.

Few consider it but putting artificial caps on your teeth will also affect your taste buds and the efficiency of your digestion. Adults with false teeth don't enjoy their food so much and not just because they are worried their teeth will break.

Another unattractive sight is that of a mouthful of dirty grey fillings. Less common these days as dentists favour almost invisible white fillings, amalgam fillings have been given a bad press because they contain mercury, which is toxic to the body. Before you rush to have them all replaced rest assured that any damage was done years ago and, according to my own dentist, you are more likely to get mercury poisoning from the fish you eat than from your fillings.

Prevention is better than cure – keep those pegs clean is the moral of this story.

Stained teeth are not the stuff of great beauty. The worst offenders for staining teeth today are coffee, tea, tobacco and red wine along with certain medications.

Teeth-whitening toothpastes are commonplace and not hugely effective. At-home whitening systems include strips that go on your teeth.

Professional tooth bleaching is increasingly popular. Dentists claim it is the fastest growing part of their business.

This is hardly surprising when you look at the improbably snowy celebrity teeth we are expected to emulate.

'Hair is the first thing. And teeth the second. Hair and teeth. A man got those two things he's got it all'

— James Brown

Other than hair transplants this is one area of cosmetic improvement that attracts as many men as women. As well it should. The days of double standards – women have to be thin and beautiful, men can be portly with yellowing teeth and thinning hair yet still be considered a good catch – are on the way out.

Well, sort of. If a man is rich enough he can still get away with looking pretty terrible and attract flocks of model-like women. Sadly this is exactly the kind of man who expects an unrealistic level of perfection from the women who surround him.

Make your choice – is it worth the pressure? If you decide it is, enjoy every treatment going and make him pay for it. Then try to get him to have those teeth fixed, please. There is little less appealing than kissing a man who has a mouthful of bad teeth.

Beware of taking your man down the path of male beauty. There is a fine line between sensible cosmetic improvement and knocking on the door of becoming a drag queen. If you find him in your make-up bag a response similar to finding him in your underwear drawer might be expected. But hey, we live in enlightened times after all.

White Fang: So cosmetic dentistry is condoned, even recommended, but how white is too white? If you are simply hoping to improve your smile, err on the side of naturalness

Cosmetic dentistry was born in the 1970s as an offshoot of restorative dentistry in which the priority was retaining or restoring the biological function of the teeth. Unsurprisingly, the aesthetic element quickly took the lead and dentists were doing work purely for the smile.

Today there is more concern about retaining the function of teeth as well as improving appearance and new materials and techniques are constantly being developed. Preserving the original tooth and doing as little damage as possible is encouraged. Still, with caps or veneers lasting on average only ten years it is a lucrative business.

– a shade or two lighter than your actual colour is enough. Accept that the older you are the less natural bright white teeth will look and stick to a subtler colour.

Before booking the appointment see a hygienist – it could be sloppy cleaning that has led to such yellowing and a power-jet of baking soda could be all you actually need.

Whiter teeth are one of the fastest ways of shaving ten years off your appearance but there is nothing that will attract ridicule as much as a middle-aged man who suddenly appears with an obviously new set of gnashers. (Different shapes and sizes are one to avoid.) Mid-life crisis springs to mind. As with all things cosmetic, less is more.

You know you have hit on the right shade of white if people start telling you how healthy you look or say things along the lines of 'you look great, something's different – have you had your hair cut?'

After all, you might be vain enough to have your teeth fixed or lightened but you don't want everyone to know that you are.

Toothbrushes – if that's what you can call a small branch or 'chew stick' – have been used since 3000 BC. The first bristle brushes were seen in China around 1500 and were made from the tough hair of a Siberian hog. Only upper-class Europeans of this time used anything to clean their teeth at all – usually an ineffective, soft horsehair brush.

The discovery of nylon by Du Pont in 1938 revolutionised the tooth-cleaning industry, providing an excellent replacement for hog hair. But the first nylon brushes were so tough that they damaged people's gums badly and were shunned by dentists. A softer nylon produced around 1950 allowed the manufacture of the toothbrush that we know today. The first electric toothbrush appeared in 1961.

Toothpaste was used by the Egyptians in 2000 BC, made from powdered pumice stone and wine vinegar. The Romans believed that urine whitened teeth!

Teeth whitening started in barbers' shops, where teeth were filed down with a metal file and finished with nitric acid. This was so corrosive that it destroyed the enamel although it was so effective at whitening teeth that it was used up until the eighteenth century.

Fluoride was used from the early part of the twentieth century but too much of it can stain teeth in later life.

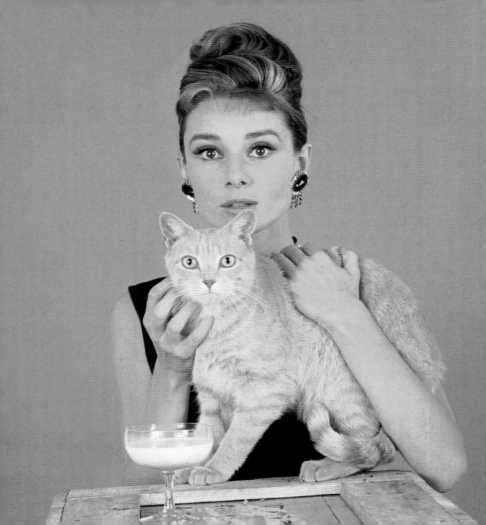

Hair-Raising Tales

'There was a little girl, who had a little curl right in the middle of her forehead...'

When hair is good it is very, very good, but when it is bad it is horrid.

'The hair is the richest ornament of women'

— Martin Luther

We all have bad hair days. Fewer and further between are good hair days. Wouldn't life be so much simpler if every day was a good hair day? Contradictory advice, on style, condition, when to wash, when not to wash, to live with natural colour or dye to change it, makes the perfect hairstyle almost impossible to find.

Accept that what suits you when you are in your teens and twenties won't necessarily suit you when you are older. The classic example being luxuriant long tresses as a girl contrasted with the straggly old hippy hair of the prematurely greying, middle-aged woman. Harsh stereotype maybe, but do take an honest look in the mirror and face facts.

Holding onto your locks is not the way to hold onto your youth. You're better off with a classic chic bob.

The exception is the chignon – the epitome of stylish hair on an older woman. This only works if you know how to pull your hair up into a chignon and don't rely on a good cut to disguise a blurred jaw-line, etc. Though the chignon is chic it is rather a waste to have long hair if you only ever wear it up.

Long, straight hair on women over 35 rarely looks good. Only Jerry Hall has got away with keeping her hair the same for thirty years without looking hopelessly out of date. Just.

When choosing a hairstyle resist cutting out a picture of your favourite celebrity from a magazine and taking it into the hairdresser saying 'I want to look like that'. This is every hairdresser's worst nightmare and puts you at a disadvantage to begin with. Better to find a hairdresser you trust – or have been recommended – and ask what he/she suggests. Have a consultation and then put yourself in their hands.

This is scary. You may well be scarred from the first time your mother took you to her hairdresser aged around 12 announcing that your scraggy, unkempt locks had to go.

Whatever the result – an unattractive bob, fluffy layering and a blow-dry that made you look about 35 or worse still a bad perm – it can take years to recover.

Similarly, if you want to have your hair coloured, don't do it yourself. It may seem like a cheaper alternative but it is a false economy. Invariably, you will have to go to a salon to have a disaster rectified and you could do damage to your hair that will take many months to recover from.

Before you balk at the cost remember teenage flirtation with bottles of Sun-In ('What do you mean, only apply two sprays, surely a whole bottle will have a better effect?!') or the subsequent turning green in the swimming pool that home-bleaching causes.

As far as colouring goes you tend to get what you pay for, so go to a good salon if you can afford it. Home (yours or theirs) colourists can be economical but be aware that they are not always in touch with the latest techniques.

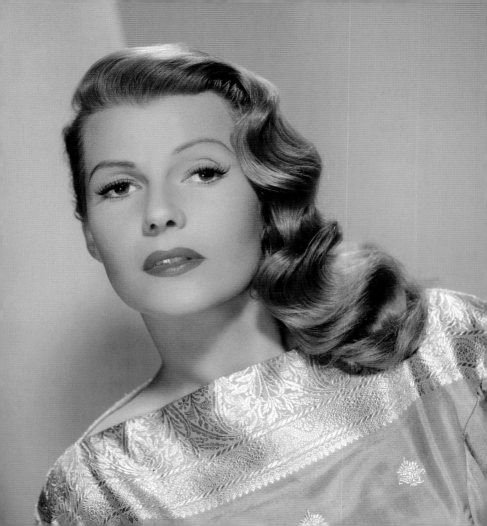

If you have made an amateur mistake or, worse still, have been turned too blonde, too dark or the wrong colour in a salon, don't panic. Most disasters can be rectified in the hands of an expert. Don't pay the culprit hairdresser. Then go and find someone who knows what they are doing. It is okay to have a cry first.

Above all, be reasonable and keep it relatively natural. If you are dark brown you can dye your hair ash blonde only for a short while before it gives up the ghost and is ruined for good. Moreover, your natural colour tends to suit your skin tone, give or take a few shades.

Skin pales with age so a colour that looks striking in your twenties will be too harsh at fifty.

Highlighting is an easier route to maintain that full head of colour, unless you are prematurely grey in which case keeping your roots up is essential for morale.

'Grey hair is a sign of age, not of wisdom'

— Greek proverb

A rough guide to styles and colours

The shape of your face and your skin tone are the two things to consider when going for a hairstyle and/or colour. A few basic tips:

Square face: A soft, longer or layered style perhaps with curls to soften a blunt-edged face shape. Part on one side, not in the middle, and avoid a square-cut fringe. Sharply defined styles will emphasise the squareness.

• 115 •

Round face: Short styles work well, particularly a short fringe or hair swept up high from the forehead to elongate it. Lots of curls are a mistake as is a scraped-back ponytail.

Hair grows at a rate of about one centimetre each month. Each hair lasts between one and six years, after which it is shed and a new hair replaces it from beneath. Around 100 hairs are lost each day. This growing phase shortens as you age, which is why it is more difficult to grow your hair longer when you are older.

Hair density also lessens with age although women are less likely to suffer from baldness than men. Your hair is thickest between the ages of 15 and 25 and thins between the ages of 30 and 50 after which the loss levels off. Loss of colour usually starts around the age of 40 but can happen far earlier.

Hormones affect the quality of hair: greasier and curlier in adolescence, drier after the menopause.

During pregnancy, hair becomes thicker because hair loss decreases with the higher levels of oestrogen and progesterone. After pregnancy, the hair that would have been lost over nine months falls out, often at an alarming rate.

Oval face: Lucky you – the best shape for hairstyles, most will look good.

Heart-shaped or widow's peak: Fringes long or short. Let the hair fall to conceal a widow's peak or part the hair in a way that makes the most of it.

Long face: Avoid long, straight hair and choose layers or a style that gives more volume at the sides. A fringe will shorten the face.

Problems including big noses, pointed chins, irregular features or an uneven hairline are best solved by a style that distracts attention from the offending feature. For example, a fringe will hide a multitude of sins from a widow's peak to a high forehead. (But though it will cover a spotty adolescent forehead contact with your equally greasy hair will not improve the condition.)

Hairstyles are all about balance. A pointed chin benefits from a wide style at the jaw, a big nose is minimised by big hair. Within reason. You don't want to make things worse than they already are.

As for colouring...

Pale skin: When you are young and porcelain-skinned you can get away with anything from pale gold to gothic black. When you are older avoid dark or intense colours.

Yellow-based skin tones: Avoid yellow or gold. Deep reds and burgundies work better.

Red faced: Rosy faces sit better with ash tones than with golden blonde or red.

Olive skins: Keep with the dark theme with warming brown, chestnut or dramatic dark brown.

Jet black hair is hard to pull off whatever your skin colour. Risking sounding in favour of the blue-rinse brigade (an aside: why do old ladies always have the same perm and colour, is there something we don't know about it?) a purple hint to jet-black hair can make a dramatic impact without washing your skin out completely.

Last but not least know your dye terminology

Permanent is not. The colour grows out, leaving roots showing, so you need to retouch every six to eight weeks.

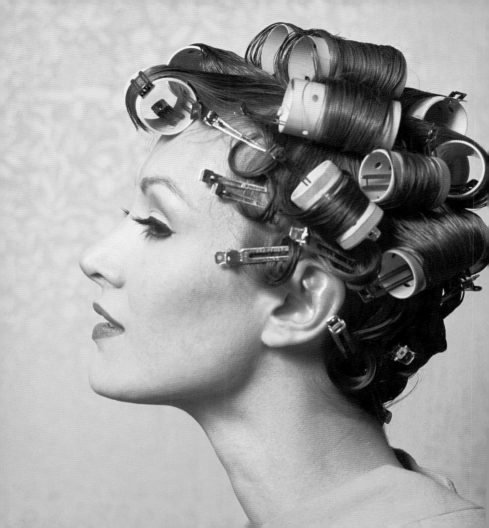

Rinse or vegetable colour only temporarily colours and will wash out within six to eight washes though it does give dull hair a lift.

Semi-permanents last longer than a rinse but not much – still expect to lose most of the colour within ten washes.

'Beauty Parlour: a place where women curl up and dye'

— Aiken Drum

Looking after your hair is as important as the style. More so, in fact. Condition buys you a lot of leeway when it comes to having beautiful hair.

Shampoo contains detergents to clean hair but may also contain preservatives including formaldehyde, common salt – added to thicken shampoo – acid such as citrus and antiseptics to control bacterial growth.

Reading the list of ingredients on your shampoo bottle seems like a good idea but the chances of you gleaning any lay information from ingredients such as lauryl sulphates (cleaning agents) or alkyl amino acids (to improve condition) are slight.

In fact, rather like reading the list of ingredients on your favourite snack it is a fast track to paranoia about what you are exposing your body to.

Basically, being sensible is the best that you can do. Try a shampoo. If it works, keep using it. If it irritates your scalp or your hair seems to look worse, change. Hairdressers often recommend changing shampoos regularly rather in the spirit of changing one's vitamin supplement as the body tends to adapt to whatever is being used on it so the product becomes less effective.

That said I have been happily using the same brand for many years and seen no ill-effects, at least I don't think so…

The theory that hair is actually self-cleaning if you give it time to re-adjust to its natural state may well be true but do you want to look as if you have had your head stuck in a bucket of lard for eight weeks to find out?

As far as hair products go great claims are made about glossy hair, pH balance and mending split ends. These really are only that – claims. But as with most things there is a degree of getting what you pay for.

Conditioners put back what shampoos take out. Absurd but true. Well, maybe not so absurd as the oil that has been washed out of your hair is teeming with dirt and pollutants.

The language of conditioners is even more complicated than that of shampoos. Perhaps because we all feel guilty about how badly we are treating our hair, manufacturers know we are sitting ducks for all kinds of promises of an easy way to perfect, glossy hair.

If only it were true.

Your bog-standard conditioner is oil suspended in an emulsion of water to create the creamy substance we know and love. More intensive conditioners may contain proteins to temporarily strengthen damaged hair, but once the damage is done no miracle can repair it.

Split-end treatments surround the broken hair with a microscopic film that supposedly repairs it. This is rubbish – it will only last until the next shampoo or brush, which will remove it.

There is only one cure for split ends: cut them off.

A strand of hair is made up of three layers: cuticle, cortex and medulla. The outer layer is made up of interlocking scales that allow things like shampoo and potentially harmful substances such as chlorine to enter the hair. They also let protein – essential for keeping hair strong – out. These scales only open to a certain width and the molecules found in cheaper shampoos are often too big, therefore cannot enter the hair.

A build-up of products such as these can damage the hair follicle – in severe cases, irreparably. Try the scratch test and see: if you run your fingernail over your scalp at the front of your head you will find a white residue – this is the legacy of years of old shampoos and styling products left unwashed away. The worse the quality of products you use the more the residue that will remain, eventually strangling the hair follicle and leading to breakages and thinner hair.

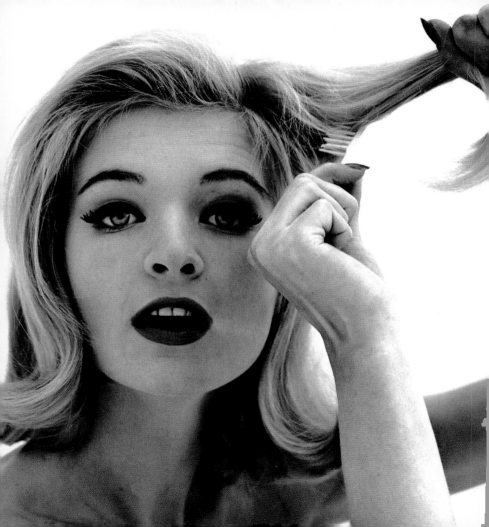

The bottom line is that there is no such thing as a miracle cure in this world – if you colour, perm, over-blow-dry, product-abuse or simply tear a comb wildly through your hair you can patch things up but not repair.

Hair is not like skin. It does not heal. So, stop expecting so much from your shampoos and conditioners. Stop spending a fortune on miracle hot-oil, leave-in, extra-strengthening products and start taking care of your hair in the first place.

Like the face – cleanse, tone, moisturise – hair needs a wash, a condition and a good styling or protective product to finish off.

How to wash your hair... PROPERLY!

First, accept that a good hair wash doesn't happen in the two and a half minutes you allow yourself in the shower each morning.

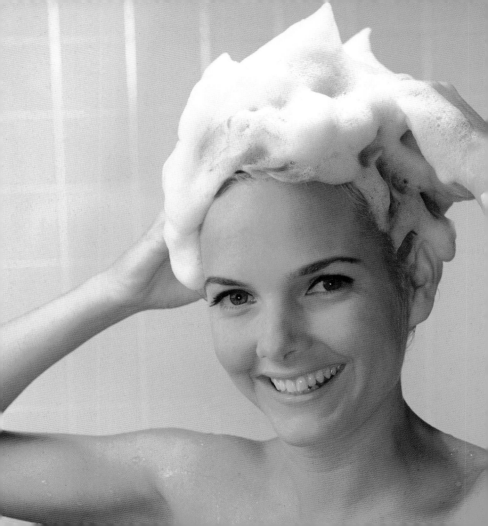

Shampoo should be used sparingly and worked into the hair for minutes, not seconds, then rinsed for at least three times longer than you think you need to rinse for. Conditioners need to be left in for as long as they say on the packet. Don't use a leave-in conditioner for a few minutes and expect the same result. Rinse and rinse again until hair feels like wet hair, not like wet hair with conditioner in it. It is surprising how many of us only feel we have conditioned hair if we can still sort of feel its presence. It has finished working, get rid of it or it will do more harm than good.

Find a range that works for you – high-quality ingredients, up-to-date research and a leaning towards more natural substances are all good pointers. Reluctant as I am to admit it, it might even pay to listen to advertising… up to a point. But be sceptical about miracle cures. There are none.

The bottom line is that a shampoo or conditioner is only that. Nothing will make your hair shine like eating a good diet, getting enough sleep and quitting your twenty-a-day cigarette habit. Similarly, drugs of any kind, prescription or otherwise, can play havoc with your hair. If you genuinely need them don't beat yourself up but otherwise ...

And have your hair cut regularly. Hair growth is stimulated by regular cutting – a bit like regular pruning of plants.

As with all things to do with beauty, nothing works so well as being in good health, and money can't buy you that.

And what about hair that is not on your head...

The pursuit of long and luxurious hair on our heads is one thing but lush hair growth can occur in places you'd rather not have it.

Depilation of hair from legs, bikini lines, underarms, forearms and faces is more common than most women are willing to admit to. We all like to perpetuate the myth that we are as hairless as the day we were born but a few weeks of letting it all go when on holiday will prove otherwise.

On a serious note, facial hair or excessive body hair can be a paralysing disfigurement for some women, so sorting it out is not so much a way of being beautiful as just feeling normal.

To shave or to wax? That is the question. Shaving is where most of us start, often too eagerly, as anyone who has felt the horrendous itching when hair starts to grow back in certain areas will know. Waxing is what we do when we have settled into a serious relationship and don't mind being hairy from time to time.

It is a myth that shaving makes hairs grow back faster than waxing. But it seems as if they do. And there is some truth in the claim that waxing makes hairs grow back softer.

· 131 ·

Everyone shaves their legs sometimes, because who is organised enough to remember to book a wax every time they want to wear a short skirt? Only the fair or lucky get away with showing off legs that are awaiting a wax. And of course you can never get a wax appointment when you have a date.

Shaving has a cultural divide. Americans shave, Europeans wax. It's just one of those things.

Shave underarms (waxing underarms is horrendously painful and as for hairy pits... in summer?!) but wax bikini lines, arms if you feel you are unduly hairy (a subject for debate, this one) and facial hair (moustaches, but not eyebrows).

Bikini lines should be just that – the line where the bikini ends. The 'landing strip' school of waxing, otherwise known as the Brazilian, was born from the teeny-tiny bikinis worn by bronzed Brazilian goddesses – the kind of women who make you reach for a kaftan before they spot your bikini, which compared to theirs resembles all the flags of the United Nations tied together.

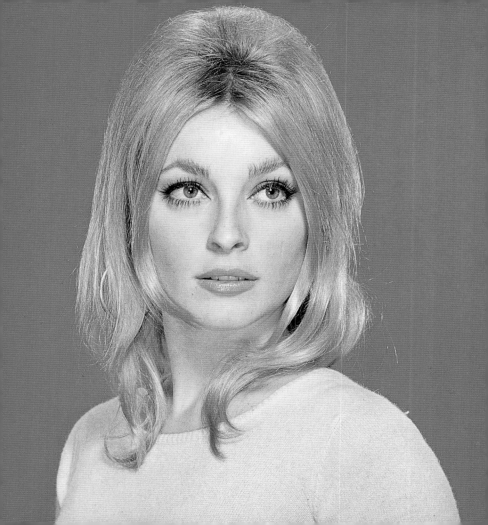

Having a Brazilian hurts. The best you can hope for is that your waxer is fast, strong and knows what she is doing.

A Hollywood takes things to new levels of nudity. All off. Rather you than me. And if your husband/boyfriend demands this (more than a novelty one-off, at least) be worried.

If you do like the look (psychoanalyst's aside: is this some kind of unwillingness to grow up?) be consoled that it always hurts most the first time you have it done.

Only models, actresses and a certain kind of 'working girl' can really justify 'needing' a Brazilian wax.

• 134 • Facial hair removal is not so much a matter of vanity but necessity for many women. There are a number of options. Tweezing is not one of them as it distorts the hair follicle and can cause real damage.

Electrolysis kills hairs over a period of time. But this can be a long time. Don't expect one course to make a huge difference. It works best on small patches of hair, rather than, for example, whole legs. If you go for a session be prepared for redness for a good few hours afterwards. Don't book an important appointment straight afterwards.

Laser depilation was pioneered for really serious cases of hirsuteness. Think of babies born looking like gorillas. Inevitably it has been hijacked by the beauty industry. A shot from a laser kills the hair root and stops re-growth. But it works on the pigmentation so if you are blonde forget it. Basically the really hairy will see a permanent difference over a few sessions. The simply vain will not.

As with all things how much hairiness is acceptable varies. A Park Avenue Princess will scream at the slightest sign of a faint blonde hair halfway up her thigh. Certain Northern Europeans will think nothing of parading a full leg of hair. Each to their own.

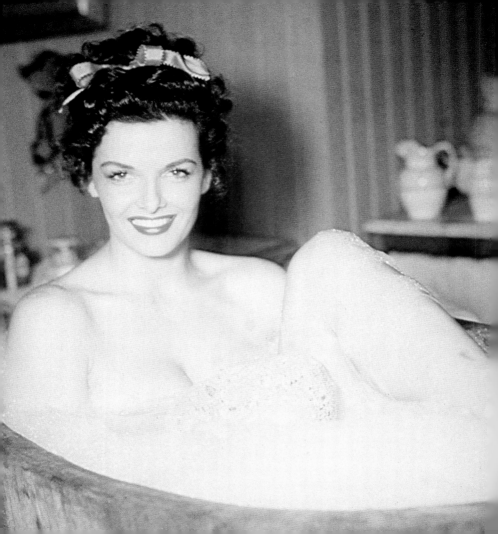

Soft as a Baby's...

If you want to look good, take care of your skin. Simple as that. Start as young as you can and keep it up. There is only so much that cosmetic camouflage can conceal and if you don't treat the canvas the paint won't look good. So if you don't know your AHAs from your antioxidants here are the basics of skincare.

Looking after your skin takes more than a quick scrub with soap and water and hoping nature will look after the rest. As skin is not created equal the first step to successful skincare is identifying whether you have oily, dry, combination or sensitive skin.

Oily skin is as it sounds, shiny, greasy and the bane of every teenage girl's (and boy's) life. Those with oily skin tend to also suffer from open pores. Interestingly, it is not only puberty that triggers this reaction in the skin but stress too. Before you get too disheartened, as you get older, oily skin suffers less from wrinkling and unsightly dry patches and offers more protection from the elements.

Don't be tempted to use harsh products, hoping to strip oil away, as you'll only make it worse. Strange as it seems, a cleansing oil (not water-based lotion) works best – like attracts like and it will draw natural oils away from the skin. Do moisturise – it won't make the problem worse – but choose a water-based one or one designed for oily skin.

Dry skin tends to be dull and flaky with rough patches, particularly across the cheeks. It is a result of the body producing too few oils. Dry skin can be a temporary effect, for example when breast-feeding a baby the essential fats in the body are diverted to milk and the skin can suffer from a lack of oil as a consequence. It is also far more common as you get older.

Use a gentle cream or wax-based cleanser (warmed between the hands for maximum effect). Oil-based moisturisers, night creams and masks work well. Avoid very hot or cold water, which will stress the skin too much.

Skin that is dry could just be an indication of overall dehydration in the body. Dehydrated skin does have oily patches, distinguishing it from dry skin. Drink plenty of water. This is universally good advice for all skin types.

Normal or combination skin. Few of us have perfectly plump, evenly toned skin but if this is the general picture of your face, congratulations. An oily T-zone, across forehead, nose and chin, is common enough to be considered normal and measures can be taken to reduce this.

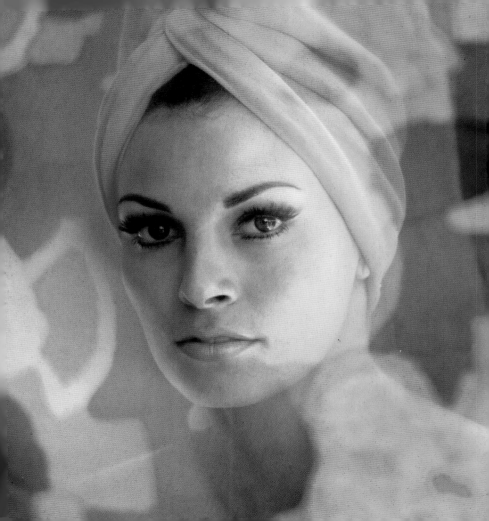

Even if you are lucky with your skin don't take it for granted and don't try and solve the T-zone problem with something akin to industrial paint stripper. Cleanse gently – a wash-off cleanser works well – and moisturise drier areas more heavily.

Sensitive skin is a word bandied about by skincare manufacturers to play on everyone's belief that their skin is so precious it needs the most delicate skincare of all. This is true in some cases but really sensitive skin is a curse, not a blessing. It is prone to redness, dryness and flaking and will develop lines and wrinkles more easily than other types. And forget sun bathing.

The golden rule is to be gentle and use the purest skincare you can find. Essential oil-based products are good. Avoid harsh exfoliants and don't experiment too much in an attempt to find the best regime. The simpler the better will help to prevent adverse reactions.

The bane of most skin types is the blackhead caused by oil hardening before it reaches the surface creating a plug that then traps dirt to create the dreaded blackhead. Although squeezing a blackhead is one of life's most satisfying experiences, try to resist. Using a metal blackhead extractor is no better. Pore-cleansing strips work to a degree, better still leave it to professionals who steam the face to loosen the blackhead and very gently (and expertly) apply pressure that miraculously extracts blackheads without scars or infection. How do they do that?

Spots are enemy number one and result when bacteria cause infection in the skin. They are worse at times of hormonal change (usually puberty) and stress when excess oil is produced. They also have an uncanny knack of appearing on important occasions... wedding days, important job interviews, etc.

Regular good skincare (combined with good diet but more of that later) will help alleviate spots. When all else fails buy a good concealer and forget about it. Other women are too preoccupied with their own appearance to notice a flaw in yours, and men are simply unobservant. If you have a real Mount Vesuvius hold your head up high and try to ignore the fact that people are talking to your chin.

Seriously though, bad acne is emotionally as well as physically disabling. It isn't true that people with acne don't look after their skins – the reverse is often true. Seeking professional help is worthwhile. Antibiotics and prescription, vitamin-A-based drugs are available and can have good results in extreme cases. In the long run it is worth trying a more holistic approach, addressing diet, lifestyle and stress management as drug treatment can have other unwanted side-effects. There are few quick fixes in this world, unfortunately.

Don't squeeze! Sorry to ruin your fun but squeezing spots spreads the bacteria, damages the skin (particularly as you

Skin is the largest organ of the body and renews itself approximately every 50 days by shedding dead skin cells.

The average adult has 2 square metres of skin, which weighs 3 kg and has approximately 300 million skin cells. It is thickest on the palms and soles of the feet and thinnest on the lips and around the eyes.

Skin is elastic, virtually waterproof, yet has oils in the top layer of the epidermis that stop water evaporating. It keeps out bacteria and guards against infection and to a certain degree attack through flexibility provided by collagen. This reduces with age as skin thins, which is why elderly skin is more fragile and damages more easily than in the young through flexibility provided by collagen, a supportive protein substance produced by the body that acts as a connective 'glue' between tissues.

get older when it doesn't repair itself so easily) and can scar. Although sometimes it is very, very hard to resist...

If you really have to squeeze, clean the area thoroughly, cover your fingertips with tissue and apply pressure on either side (NOT with your nails, but with your tips). A spot of blood (sorry to be blunt) indicates the offender is out, dab with tea-tree oil, which is a natural disinfectant, and LEAVE WELL ALONE.

Cleanse, tone, moisturise... the mantra of beauty experts everywhere. Drill it into your daughters as young as you can and they will thank you for ever.

Once you have identified your skin type find a routine that will suit it. The basic rules are the same. Cleansing is the • 145 • most important.

How to cleanse: To remove make-up use a cream cleanser. Warm it in your hands first to emulsify it and work it thoroughly into your face with your fingers, not with cotton wool, which can be too abrasive. Removing with water prevents damage to the skin and feels refreshing at the same time. Soak a cloth in warm (not very hot) water and some lavender oil for its antibacterial properties (note: never use an essential oil neat on skin or you will burn – these oils may be natural but are also potent) and remove gently. There is something slightly grubby about not actually washing your face clean. Ignore sceptics who say water dries out your skin. What's moisturiser for, anyway?

A scrub-based cleanser (often used following a cream) is misleading because the last thing you should do is scrub. Gently press into the face, particularly your T-zone, with your fingertips. The aim is to create a kind of suction that pulls the deep dirt out, not to remove the entire top layer of your skin. Scrubbing yourself raw may feel beneficial but the trend for harsh skincare went out with the carbolic soap during the Second World War, bar the no-nonsense approach of few old-fashioned English nannies.

Toner is designed to tighten it all up again. Again, applying with cotton wool is too harsh. A spray toner that you gently pat into the skin and allow to dry naturally works best. Don't be tempted by overly astringent versions. Forget no pain, no gain. If it stings it means it's too harsh, not that it is working.

Moisturising is an area of contradictions. Some facial experts believe that skin becomes lazy if you give it too much help with a moisturiser, preferring to cleanse the skin and leave it (often overnight, allowing a light moisturiser during the day) to rebalance itself. In theory this sounds good, after all a skin should have enough natural oil to moisturise itself. But in practice skin can feel very tight if no moisturiser is used.

Advocates of the leaving it alone regime say that this will rebalance over time but those who love the feel of a rich night cream may not agree. Rather like the theory that hair will clean itself if you don't shampoo it for so many weeks, suffering mask-like skin that feels as if it can crack at any moment is no fun. Suffer tightness for a night and if, in the morning, your skin is soft and plump again with no sign of dryness you are probably okay – and will save a fortune in expensive night creams.

On balance (and that is what you want your skin to achieve) most skin types do well with a light cream at night and in summer and a heavier, more protective one during the day, mostly during the winter months when cold and wind can play havoc with skin.

Regrettably, not only do you need a different set of make-up during the summer and winter months but you need to alter your skincare regime accordingly too. Look at it logically. In summer you are sweatier, oilier and generally less exposed to harsh wind and rain. So you need a much lighter moisturiser, preferably with a sun-block.

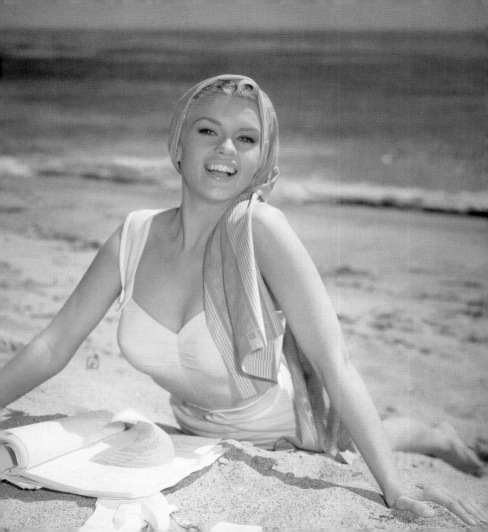

The weather is an enemy of good skin. Sun, wind, cold, heat, you name it. Only rain-water might do it some good. Picture the classic ruddy cheeks of a confirmed countrywoman, indeed the rugged complexion of any outdoor folk – lumberjacks, fishermen, etc. (Of course this is rather attractive on a man but disastrous on women. Double standards apply everywhere.)

As well as moisturisers and sun-block, make-up itself can be a good protection against the elements. Joan Collins swears that her (improbably) perfect complexion is down to wearing foundation every day of her life. She has a point. It will protect you to a certain degree.

Sun protection

Ninety per cent of skin ageing is caused by sun damage. Still tempted to ignore tan warnings? It causes liver spots, broken blood vessels, thinning of the dermis – the inner layer of skin – and wrinkling. So use a sunscreen. A moisturiser with built-in sun-block works best – always buy one designed for the face. Slapping on a generic factor 30 will work but a white face (as in covered in zinc oxide, much like white paint really) isn't really a great look.

Controversially speaking it isn't necessary to wear sun-block all year round (not in British climes at least) or even daily in summer if you only spend half an hour outside walking to and from your office.

In your working life you are more likely to suffer from air-conditioning (or, in winter, central heating). Going from hot, humid streets to unnaturally cold and dry offices, throwing in a dose of urban pollution along the way and no wonder your skin suffers.

Be sensible. Sun-block may protect you from the sun but the chemicals (or even naturally found minerals in 'healthy' ones) may take their own toll. And they tend to be greasy and pore-clogging. Stay out of the sun between

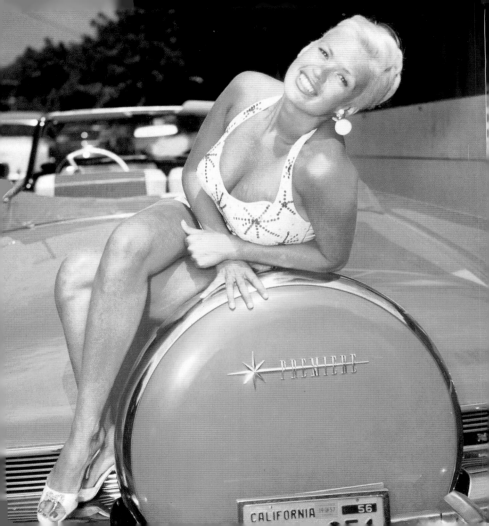

11 a.m. and 3 p.m., sit in the shade, wear a hat and when you do want to enjoy some gentle sunshine, then apply your screen.

You know what they say about mad dogs and Englishmen...

Some other tempting promises of rejuvenation...

Anti-ageing (or anti-wrinkle) creams are big business, playing on our insecurities as usual, but outrageous claims may be on their way out. Research shows that the more a cream claims to be able to 'reverse the signs of ageing' the less likely we are to believe it. Consumers are not so stupid after all, it seems. It is better to buy none, however, than buy cheap. The (mostly unproven, but probably effective) raw ingredients don't come cheap, so up to a point you do get what you pay for.

This 'get what you pay for' maxim is pretty much true when it comes to cosmetic creams, galling as it sounds. But console yourself that you don't need the whole range; a cleanser and moisturiser are the most important. The rest are mostly retailer add-ons.

Eye creams are even more expensive per drop than night creams. Fortunately, the area around the eye is proportionately tiny. The skin is thinnest and most vulnerable around the eyes so a cream is worth investing in but less is more; you only need a tiny amount so don't waste the stuff. And try justifying a £50-plus pot the size of your thumbnail to the man in your life (sorry, very non-feminist, to yourself then) more than once every six months.

- 154 - Day creams and night creams are just a way of making you spend more money. Unless you have pots of the stuff (money, not cream) an all-rounder will do.

Masks come in all different guises for different skin types. The best cleanse gently and deeply and can be used regularly. The worst peel off half your face. Resign yourself to the fact that your skin always looks worse for a while after a face pack, something to do with drawing out the toxins (hmm, that old chestnut) as you rush to buy more potions to rectify the damage.

Never answer the door when wearing a face mask, it could be anyone... and have you ever tried flirting with a face of green cement? As for smiling or laughing... your skin will resemble a cracked river bed after a particularly dry summer.

Professional facials will always be better than something you do at home (warning: choose your facialist with care; a bad facial is far more damaging than a bad haircut). • 155 •

You are given time, expertise and generous portions of products that would cost you far more to buy than the cost of the facial. An expert will squeeze spots without damaging skin and diagnose and advise on problems from acne to dry patches. Worth every penny if only as a pampering exercise and an excuse to look after number one for an hour or so.

What's the alternative?

Arnica is wonderful for lessening dark circles under eyes. Calendula cream is a perfect moisturiser for sensitive or eczema-prone skins. Lavender essential oil has anti-bacterial properties and tea-tree oil is a powerful natural disinfectant – dab (diluted!) on spots, particularly if you have given in and squeezed them.

And for the famed kitchen beauty regime...

If you can cope with mess and are not too tempted to eat them instead, avocado makes a good face-pack (though it turns an unattractive grey colour), cucumber or cold green tea-bags reduce puffiness around the eyes and oatmeal cleanses the skin.

None of these are as effective as professional products or, better still, salon treatments. Best to get skincare experimentation out of your system as a teenager along with home-spun attempts at hair colouring.

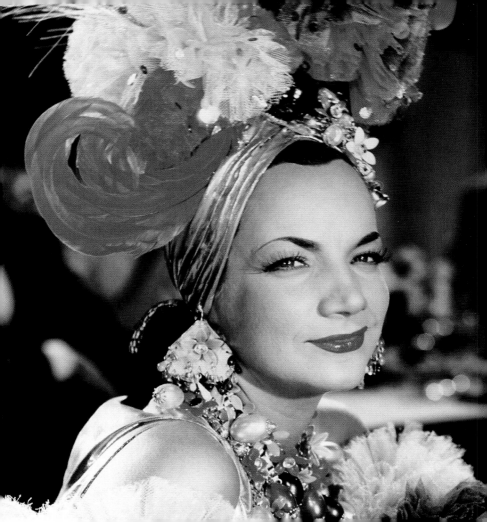

Inside Out

'I'm tired of all this nonsense about beauty being only skin-deep. That's deep enough. What do you want — an adorable pancreas?'

— Jean Kerr

Beauty may only be skin deep but if you want to be really beautiful there is only so much you can do from the outside. Paying as much – if not more – attention to what you put in, rather than on, your body is the true secret to being beautiful.

Food and drink

'Champagne is the only wine a woman can drink and still remain beautiful'

— Sophia Loren

It is time to face facts. There is no product that will make you beautiful as much as looking after yourself. What you eat and drink has a far-reaching effect on how you look and how you feel. And beauty isn't just about looks but about energy and vitality so (don't groan) it is time to re-think your lifestyle.

The answer is simple: eat well, drink plenty of water, sleep enough and avoid stress. Ha. Do we live in the modern world or what?

Okay. But at least try.

The best beauty foods (that taste good too...)

Best for skin:

For plumpness: Fat! Hurrah! But before you reach for the deep fryer it has to be the right kind. Mono- or poly-unsaturated with an emphasis on essential fatty acids. Don't balk at the jargon. Think avocados, nuts and seeds and oily fish like salmon and sardines. All good for plumpness and smoothness. Collagen and elastin, a similar protein that is the main constituent of elastic tissues in the body, are also enhanced by fruits including berries. Strawberries and cream (full-fat milk products are the ones with most vitamins, hurrah!) all round, please.

For youthful skin: Anti-oxidant-rich foods. Fruit and vegetables that are colourful – think red (tomatoes, peppers), orange (mangoes, papayas, sweet potatoes) and green (asparagus, broccoli). Also wholemeal grains: bread, rice, rye. Anti-oxidant-rich foods also counter the effects of ultra-violet rays.

Anti-ageing: Antioxidants as above and also soya-based foods that aid regeneration and slow down the ageing process: soya milk, tofu and soya yoghurt. Seaweed is also reputed to help skin renewal.

Don't eat any of these if you really don't like them. A sour-taste face is not a pretty one. If you claim you don't like any of these foods give up on looking glowingly beautiful right now. A diet of processed food is the path to sallow, pasty, spotty skin that no cosmetics will make look any better.

Acne can be helped with vitamin-A-rich foods. The best is betacarotene (found in orange fruit and vegetables such as carrots), which the body converts as it needs, rather than the vitamin A found in meats such as liver, which can be toxic if over-consumed.

Eczema and psoriasis benefit from essential fatty acids found in nuts and seeds and oily fish as well as evening primrose oil, which can reduce itching and inflammation.

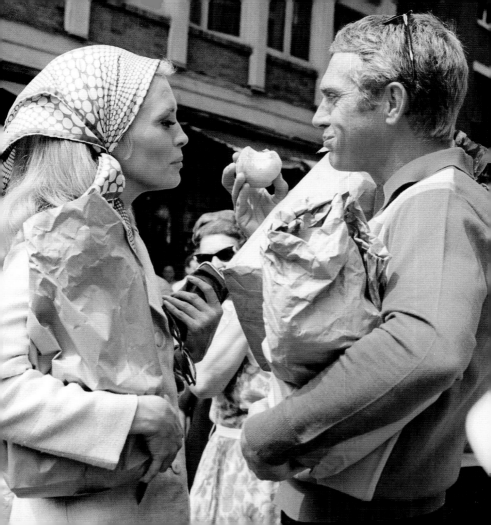

DRINK WATER!

Lots. To be precise at least one and a half to two litres a day, minimum. And an extra glass for every glass of wine and cup of coffee, if you are exercising, breast-feeding or it is very, very hot. Carry it with you for ease.

Do remember that with all things it is possible to overdose on water. In very hot climates paranoid water-guzzlers commonly flush all the salt out of their bodies, causing them to collapse, and kidney strain can occur if you drink too much water. Listen to your body but remember that by the time you feel thirsty you are already dehydrated.

Hydrating foods include watermelon, celery and cucumber.

Best for nails: Nails need calcium and silicon found in dairy products but also in sardines, nuts and seeds (particularly sesame), eggs and oats. Good circulation is also important and is promoted by garlic, ginger and gingko biloba.

White flecks are caused by a zinc deficiency. By far and away the highest level of zinc is found in oysters. Also an aphrodisiac if the thought of a slippery hors d'oeuvre is too much for you.

DRINK WATER... to stop brittleness and keep nails from drying out.

Best for hair: Golden rule – don't diet. Double hurrah! Well, not crash dieting. Hair is one of the first places that nutrient deficiencies show up. Iron is essential to encourage growth (eat red meat, dark green vegetables, dried fruit) as are omega-3 essential fatty acids (oily fish, almonds, flax seeds).

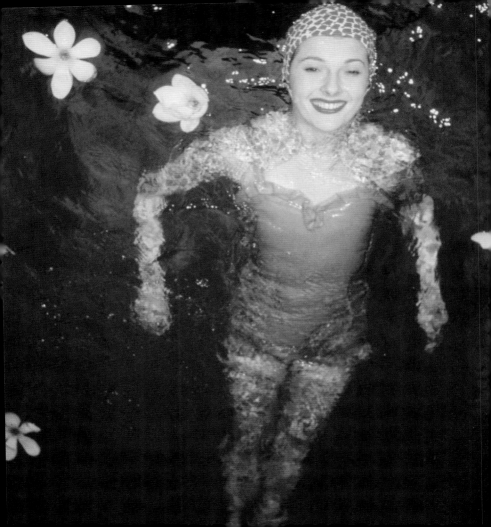

Growth-promoting foods that help maintain strong hair are iodine-rich. Seaweed is the richest source. Good-quality protein (fish, lean meat) is also essential for keratin, which coats hair and keeps it strong.

DRINK WATER to make sure hair stays healthy and glossy.

Avoid stress: Try St John's wort (nicknamed the natural Prozac) and get enough sleep with chamomile tea before bed.

Eat natural food: It always seems to make sense to eat food that is as un-tampered-with and unprocessed as possible as presumably your body knows what to do with it. Not just health foods, the nice stuff too. Think butter, not margarine.

Chocolate has plenty of magnesium in it, in case you needed justification (only the 70% cocoa stuff, though!)

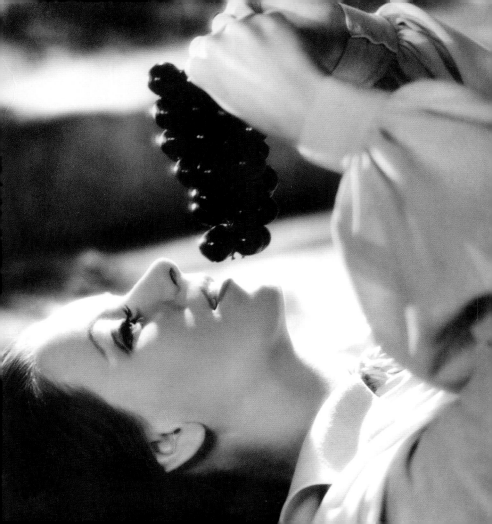

Caffeine is not so good (and chocolate has plenty of that too) but coffee is worse than tea which Asian systems of health positively advocate.

Avoid toxins: Yes, that means all the usual suspects, caffeine, alcohol, additives, drugs, prescription or otherwise. It may be worth investigating problem foods such as dairy products, excess sugar or yeast, although getting to the bottom of food allergies is a marathon effort that is more often subject to fashion than scientific fact.

All things in moderation sounds old-fashioned but is the best advice. Extreme diets or de-toxes place a great strain on the body. So eat a wide variety of foods (to get a variety of nutrients) and have a few squares of chocolate or a glass of wine. (If you do clean up your diet expect problems like skin to get worse before they get better, that old toxins coming out thing again...)

To counter ill-effects from anything you over-indulge in (that will show up first in dry/greasy or spotty skin, dull eyes, lank hair, etc.) DRINK WATER... Sorry, did I say that, already?

And another excuse to pamper yourself...

Massage improves circulation, reduces stress and works wonders on poor skin tone. Consider regular treatments an essential part of your beauty regime – far more cost-effective than the latest miracle anti-cellulite cream.

The best massages

Deep tissue: The hard school of pummelling, treating your body like a gristly steak that needs plenty of tenderising. Good for getting rid of knots and tension.

Swedish: Similarly invigorating – preferably administered by a stern European blonde with impossibly strong hands.

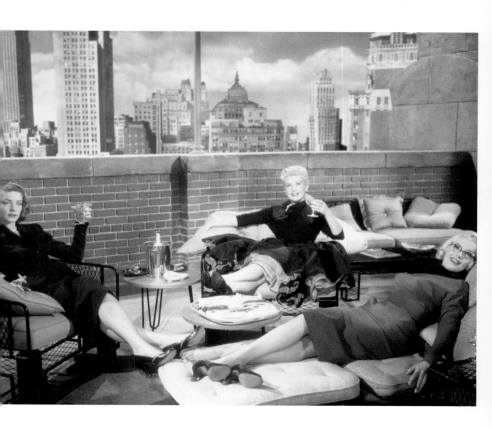

Thai, Balinese, Ayurvedic: Differing Eastern techniques that energise and cleanse. More relaxing and sometimes performed clothed.

Shiatsu: A particularly effective technique that works on the body's meridians and pressure points. Performed fully clothed and as refreshing for the mind as it is for the body.

And last but not least... Live your life, make friends, take lovers, travel, work, party, whatever turns you on... even if it means not looking perfect all the time.

'There is no cosmetic for beauty like happiness'

— Helen Rowland

A Chemical World

Having dictated that the best way to make yourself look beautiful is to care about what goes inside you, making it as natural and unpolluted as possible, it is worth scaring you into making some changes when you look at the damage everyday chemicals and pollutants do to your skin.

Cosmetics and skincare are particular culprits and though vanity tends to win hands down when you want the perfectly made-up face it is worth investigating make-up that doesn't use chemicals. This is easier said than done. Look for genuinely pure brands such as Jurlique and Dr Hauschka. Base products such as foundations and powders that leach their ingredients into your pores daily are worth changing.

Fact: women swallow on average 2–5 kg of lipstick over a lifetime.

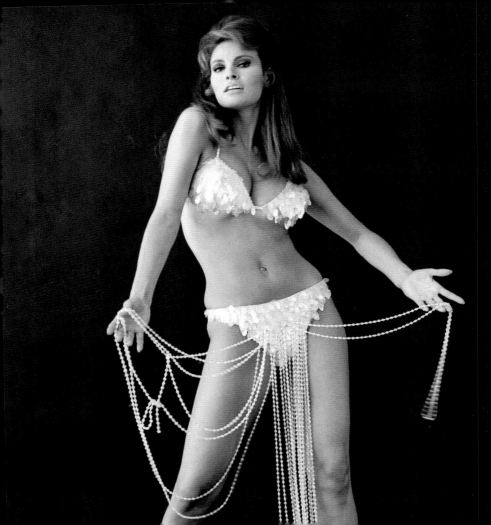

The Body Beautiful

*'It takes more than just a good-looking body.
You've got to have the heart and soul to go with it'*

— Lee Haney

When you think of a woman who is beautiful you think first of her face. But more of us obsess over the pursuit of the body beautiful than anything else.

Ask any woman which she would rather be: thin or beautiful? Sadly the answer is often the former. But

Throughout history the desirable shape for a female body has changed. Until the last century one thing remained common: plumpness was prized. Take one look at the paintings of Rubens, Renoir and Titian and see varying degrees of full flesh on thighs, stomachs and breasts, depending on the fashion of the time. It is only since the turn of the twentieth century and the start of the emancipation of women in the 1920s that women have aspired to being thin. Part of the pursuit of thinness is based on exclusivity. Until the twentieth century being fat represented wealth and status. In the twenty-first century it is more likely to be an indicator of poverty and usually of ill not good health.

consider the haggard, drawn face of the woman who has neglected her looks in pursuit of thinness and you might change your mind.

The bottom (pert, plump, flat, wide or drooping) line: thin doesn't always equal beautiful. And you'd be surprised how many of us forget that our face and body are part of the same person.

Thin people concentrate on the width of their hips and ignore sallow skin and hollow cheeks. Big women often concentrate on making their face look stunning with perfect make-up but shroud the rest of themselves in shapeless clothes. Neither of these approaches works.

A brief history of dieting madness...   • 177 •

1918 The word 'calorie' emerges from scientific circles to mainstream usage.

1920s Flapper dresses demand skinny frames and emancipation gives way to emaciation. The Hay method of food combining is born, still popular today.

1930s The Hollywood diet appears. Grapefruit becomes a girl's best friend. Certain foods are claimed to have 'negative calories', for example celery, because they use up more energy digesting than they provide.

1940–1950 Ideal weight charts appear and amphetamine-based diet drugs are all the range, side-effects notwithstanding.

1960s Weightwatchers is founded and Dr Atkins first appears on the scene. Controversy over high-protein diet rages as it still does today.

1970s Low fat, high fibre emerges. 'F'-plan groupies propel themselves windily to a slimmer self. Hippy health-food mania and vegetarianism abound. For those who

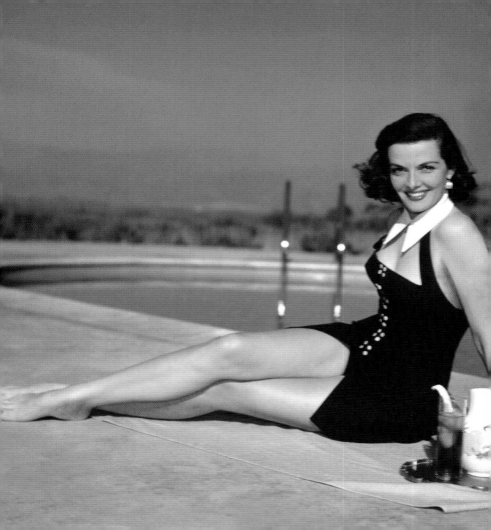

prefer quick-fix drugs, fenfluramine, the appetite suppressant, is introduced.

1980s The era of shoulder pads, Jane Fonda 'no pain, no gain' aerobics and the Beverly Hills diet. The Glycaemic Index of foods is drawn up to combat diabetes, now believed to help weight control through insulin management in all of us.

1990–2000 and onwards. Diet pill scare-mongering as links to heart problems lead to withdrawal of popular brands. Atkins reborn. Dieters embrace bacon breakfasts and bad breath in an effort to outsmart the body into slenderness. Celebrities swear by it and other similar high-protein diets. Health experts warn us of the consequences to our hearts and livers and yet still we get fatter and fatter…

Dieting doesn't work – at least not in the long term. It makes you miserable, obsessive, poor (the diet industry is a multi-billion dollar one) and ultimately fat.

So don't bother. It's boring to say it but eating healthily (see above) and taking a bit of exercise will make your body settle into a shape that suits it. And settling into what suits your body is ultimately what makes you beautiful. If you are not designed to be thin you will look ill if you lose too much weight. What is beautiful for you isn't necessarily what is beautiful for Kate Moss (who, incidentally has blossomed since the birth of a child with the extra curves that go along with motherhood).

Don't…

Count calories or go on the latest new gimmicky diet. Life is too short and your body is probably confused enough as it is.

Compare yourself to models, actresses or your super-skinny best friend.

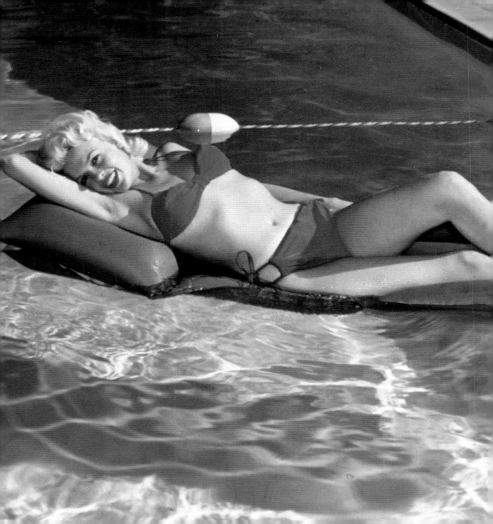

Think you can stuff yourself with something just because it is allowed on a diet plan, particularly if you don't even like it.

Get obsessive. No one likes a diet bore.

Get self-righteous if you do lose weight. You'll be eating (sorry) your words when you regain it.

Care if you do put on a little weight. Give and take is normal. Weighing yourself five times a day is not. In fact, don't bother weighing yourself. Better to be aware of the fit of your clothes, unless you favour the big and baggy, hide a few extra stone approach.

Do...

Eat healthy food you enjoy and savour quality over quantity.

Look at your face as well as your body – the two are not separate entities.

Take yourself to an exhibition of Rubens or Renoir paintings and console yourself that you were just born in the wrong century and are in fact devastatingly beautiful.

Pamper yourself. A looked-after body is a happy one, so spend your money on massages or treatments like reflexology not another diet book.

Remember a little of what you enjoy is a good thing.

A body will not be beautiful unless its owner is happy with it. Torturing yourself through diet and exercise you hate will only make you miserable and that will show on your face, in your posture and in your general daily crankiness. None of which is attractive.

Exercise is good for you. Again, boring but true that a fit

(or at least fit-ish) body is more beautiful than one that spends its life in the car. Also, you'll feel better so you'll look better. And as the body is designed to be functional it makes sense that a well-functioning body is an attractive one. But don't torture yourself. If you hate the gym go for a walk in the park.

'I'm not into working out. My philosophy: No pain, no pain'

— George H. Mead

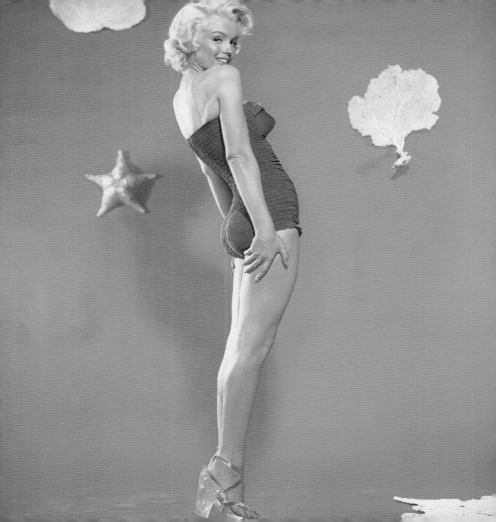

A Little Help from Our Friends – Cosmetic Surgery and the Rest…

'The most common error made in matters of appearance is the belief that one should disdain the superficial and let the true beauty of one's soul shine through. If there are places on your body where this is a possibility, you are not attractive — you are leaking'

— Fran Lebowitz

Plastic surgery became more prevalent at the end of the First World War when soldiers with shattered faces were given reconstructive surgery. Inevitably, advancements in techniques made cosmetic surgery a fast-growing area.

In the 1920s actresses began improving their facial features with techniques such as the 'bobbing' of noses. Early face-lifts were also tried, not always with great success. By the 1960s cosmetic surgery had entered the mainstream consciousness of America and by the beginning of the twenty-first century the number of people having cosmetic surgery annually ran into millions.

The danger today is where we go from here. The taboo that made women deny their surgeries (and keep them within reason) is lifting and surgery (both good and bad) is becoming available to the masses.

Sometimes it feels as if we are fighting a losing battle. It isn't enough to look after your skin, eat healthily, exercise and learn to apply cosmetics as expertly as a make-up artist. Now we are expected to compete with a entirely different class of woman – one who cheats.

I'll presume you don't rely on your looks for your income – for example, are a model or actress of the impossibly perfect Hollywood type – and urge you to stand up against the tide of cosmetic surgery.

Cosmetic surgery is everywhere. Botox at Boots in your lunch-break, face-lifts advertised on the bus, immobile breasts in bikinis on the beach, it is becoming easier to change your features than it is to correct your teeth.

But at the risk of sounding old-fashioned, why would you want to have surgery (with all its risks) when you don't actually need it? And don't say you do – the bags under your eyes can't be that bad. (Always reserve the right to change your mind once you hit sixty!)

And it seems that it is a slippery slope. Convince yourself a shot of Botox is okay, then a little eye-lift or tummy tuck and before you know it you're on your way to a full body transplant. Might as well have a personality bypass to go with it.

Across the pond: There is definitely a difference in the way Americans and Brits view plastic surgery. Americans are very open to it. The British tend not to be (or maybe they just won't admit it). Something to do with the English sense of self-deprecation and horror of appearing to be vain in any way. No stiff upper lip (or forehead) for me, thank you.

Americans on the other hand see nothing wrong in improving yourself in any way possible and bragging about it into the bargain. Having said that, there is nothing worse than the actress who condemns surgery openly then sneaks into her plastic surgeon wearing a wig, hoping no one will ever guess when she appears with eyes 50 per cent wider than they used to be.

This divide is beginning to narrow.

The lunch-time lift (or when is cosmetic improvement not surgery?)

Botox and collagen have become halfway houses for women who are too afraid to face the knife. Quite frankly, an injection of botulin is just as scary. Collagen, a cartilage derived from cows that is injected to plump out wrinkles and enhance lips, is also terrifying sounding. The thought of some cow protein injected into your mouth puts a whole new spin on the benefits of eating a fillet steak.

Laser treatments are used to remove wrinkles, brown spots, scars, stretch marks, broken blood vessels and hair.

Some burn (ablative) which can be dangerous and take two to three months to heal properly (once new skin has grown in). Others (non-ablative) are gentler and take place over a series of sessions.

Microdermabrasion or acid peels do literally that – peel away the top (or more than that) layer of skin. Think sandblasting your face.

This last technique is for repairing damaged skin. Try not damaging it in the first place. Stay out of the sun, eat well, drink lots of water and look after your skin. Then you might be a real, not artificial beauty.

And as for the body – tummy tucks, liposuction, breast implants... The list of improvements is endless and once you have started the temptation is to carry on. Take Michael Jackson as a warning...

Reasons not to have cosmetic surgery

It might go wrong! (Could there be a better reason?) And disfigurement could be the least of your worries as we read another horror story about a charlatan doctor causing death on the operating table.

Cost (NEVER try to find a bargain basement surgeon – see above).

Embarrassment. It is a Catch-22 situation. If you admit you have had it you look vain; if you deny treatment you look vain and naïve for thinking that people won't notice.

Reasons to have cosmetic surgery

Genuine physical disfigurement through birth, illness or accident.

If you feel your big nose, small breasts, etc are really a barrier to enjoying everyday life, visit a psychiatrist before booking a surgeon.

In the end you make your own decision but think hard before you decide to go under the knife.

Fear of ageing is one of the commonest reasons for seeking cosmetic surgery. We live in a world where sixty-year-old actresses are expected to appear twenty years younger (and the same goes for forty-year-old ones!). And these women are held up as our role models. No wonder we are all so paranoid.

Controversial, but maybe growing older has its own beauty if any of us were brave enough to find out.

'As a white candle
In a holy place,
So is the beauty
Of an aged face'

— Joseph Campbell

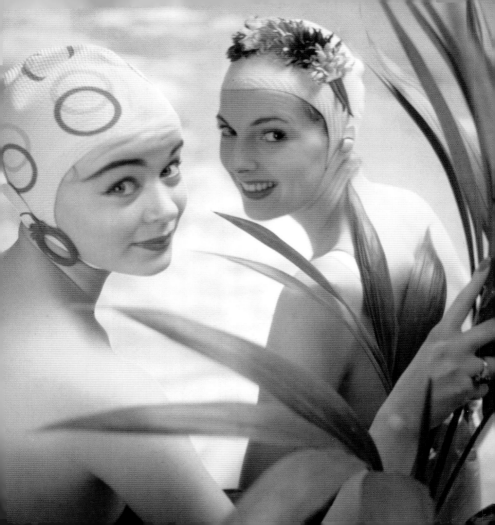

What *Really* Makes Us Beautiful Anyway...

'There is certainly no absolute standard of beauty. That precisely is what makes its pursuit so interesting'

— John Kenneth Galbraith

This book has discussed how to make yourself look and feel your best, which is about as much as anyone can hope for. Every woman has her own beauty, even if it isn't the commercial kind. Models can look peculiarly ugly at the same time as representing what is supposed to be beautiful which makes a mockery of what beauty actually is. It truly is in the eye of the beholder.

Being happy in yourself, settling into your features, your body and your life is what we should aspire to, and ultimately living is far more enjoyable and attractive than simply appearing. After all beauty can be as much of a curse as a blessing…

'Beauty is a short-lived tyranny'

— Immermann

'Beauty is worse than wine, it intoxicates both the holder and beholder'

— Kahlil Gibran

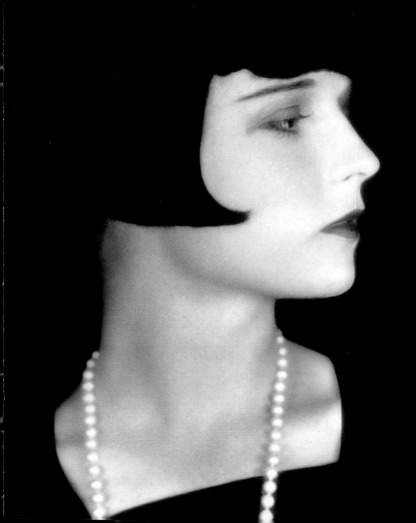

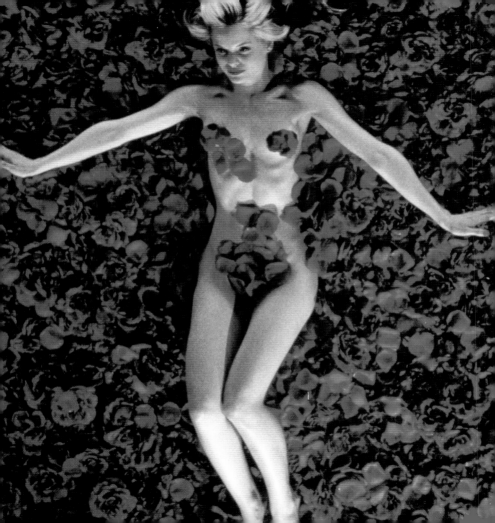

'If you're considered a beauty, it's hard to be accepted doing anything but standing around'

— Cybil Shepard

It might make an impression at first sight but it won't necessarily carry you much further than that...

'Beauty is all very well at first sight; but who ever looks at it when it has been in the house three days?'

— George Bernard Shaw

'She was a beauty in her youth a fact which she alone remembers'

— Benjamin Constant

If it catches you a lover it won't guarantee to keep him...

What *Really* Makes Us Beautiful Anyway…

> '*Beauty soon grows familiar to the lover, fades in his eye, and palls upon the sense*'
>
> — Joseph Addison

Because, clichéd as it sounds, true beauty comes from within…

> '*People are like stained glass windows — the true beauty can be seen only when there is light from within. The darker the night, the brighter the windows*'
>
> — Elizabeth Kubler-Ross

'True beauty dwells in deep retreats,
Whose veil is unremoved,
Till heart with heart in concord beats,
And the lover is beloved'

— William Wordsworth

And no cosmetics, dieting or surgery will make you attractive if you are, deep down, an ugly person. Now doesn't that make you feel better about all those Queen Bee bitches you were at school with?!

'Beauty is only skin deep, but ugly goes clear to
the bone '

— Anonymous

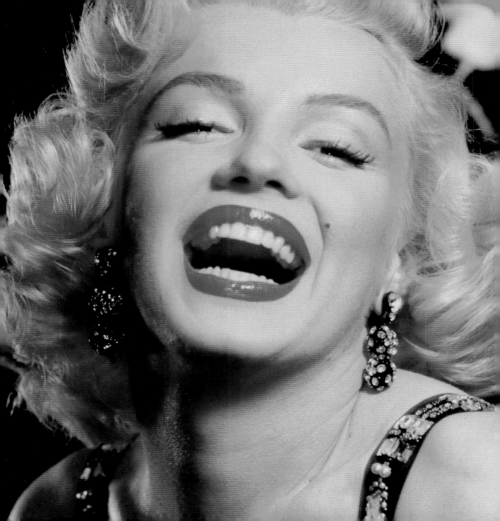

Picture Credits

The publishers would like to thank the following sources for their kind permission to reproduce the pictures in this book.

Aquarius Collection: 32

Condé Nast Publications Ltd: Clifford Coffin/Vogue: 68

Corbis Images: Genevieve Naylor: 89

Getty Images: George Fresten/Stringer: 40; /Hulton Archive: 79, 92, 128, 166, 196; /The Image Bank: 120

Picture Desk: The Kobal Collection: 21, 36, 56, 133, 149, 179, 186, 199, 204; /20th Century Fox: 5, 12, 158, 171, 174; /Bob Coburn: 113; /Columbia/Bob Coburn: 96; /Dreamworks/Jinks/Cohen/Lorey Sebastian: 200; /John Engstead: 49; /MGM: 168; /MGM/7ARTS: 84; /Paramount: 45, 74-75, 108, 136; /United Artists: 163; /Universal: 63

Rex Features: Everett Collection: 28; /Globe Photos Inc: 25, 53, 140; /SNAP: 182; /Sipa Press: 152

V&A Images: John French: 46, 126

Every effort has been made to acknowledge correctly and contact the source and/or copyright holder of each picture and Carlton Books Limited apologises for any unintentional errors or omissions that will be corrected in future editions of this book.